AF380430

M. Kusano, S. Shioda (Eds.)

New Frontiers in Regenerative Medicine

M. Kusano, S. Shioda (Eds.)

New Frontiers in Regenerative Medicine

With 44 Figures, Including 4 in Color

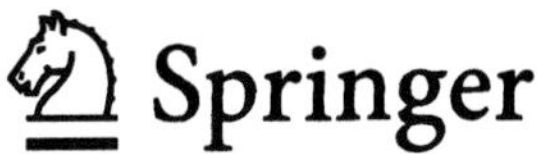 Springer

Mitsuo Kusano, MD, PhD
Professor of Surgery, Showa University School of Medicine
1-5-5 Hatanodai, Shinagawa-ku, Tokyo 142-8555, Japan

Seiji Shioda, MD, PhD
Professor of Anatomy, Showa University School of Medicine
1-5-5 Hatanodai, Shinagawa-ku, Tokyo 142-8555, Japan

Library of Congress Control Number: 2006938397

ISBN-10 4-431-38207-0 Springer Tokyo Berlin Heidelberg New York
ISBN-13 978-4-431-38207-2 Springer Tokyo Berlin Heidelberg New York

Springer is a part of Springer Science+Business Media
springer.com
© Springer 2007

Typesetting: Camera-ready by the editors and authors

Printed on acid-free paper

Foreword

It gives me great pleasure that New Frontiers in Regenerative Medicine is being published. This is a memorable book for Showa University, with much of the volume's content stemming from presentations made at the Second International Symposium for Life Sciences, held at Showa University in 2005. This symposium was supported in part by the Special Subsidies (Grants for the Promotion of the Advancement of Education and Research in Graduate Schools) funding for ordinary expenses of private schools, made available by the Ministry of Education, Culture, Sports, Science and Technology, Japan.

On behalf of Showa University, it is a privilege to present this book of research findings that advance the field of knowledge of regenerative medicine and tissue engineering. I hope that through the information presented here many physicians and surgeons of the twenty-first century will possess more powerful tools to work with regenerative medicine to find cures for a great many patients.

Akiyoshi Hosoyamada, MD, PhD
President
Showa University, Tokyo
September 2006

Preface

This book examines many of the unresolved problems as well as future applications of regenerative medicine. In the first chapter, we focus on the digestive and integumentary system, dealing with hepatocyte transplantation, pancreatic regeneration, and skin and hair regeneration. The second chapter deals with the cardiovascular system, with repair and remodeling of the lung and heart, arterial remodeling with bone marrow-derived progenitor cells, and induction of angiogenesis by adhesion molecules. The third chapter concerns the nervous system and hippocampal neurogenesis, along with the functional significance of pro-inflammatory cytokines, pituitary adenylate cyclase-activating polypeptide, and the production of free radicals after brain ischemia. In addition to animal experiments, this book includes the results of research on human tissues and organs.

Rapid advances in stem cell biology have raised exciting possibilities of replacing damaged or lost tissues and cells by activation of in vitro-expanded stem cells or their progeny. We need to identify the sources of stem cells, to understand mechanisms regulating their proliferation, fate, and, most importantly in the case of neuronal lineages, to characterize their functional properties. In addition, this volume contains material from the Showa University International Symposium for Life Sciences, held at Showa University, Tokyo, in September 2005.

This project was supported in part by a grant for The Promotion and Mutual Aid Cooperation for Private Schools of Japan and Ministry of Education, Culture, Sports, Science and Technology of Japan.

Mitsuo Kusano, Professor of Surgery, MD, PhD
Seiji Shioda, Professor of Anatomy, MD, PhD
Showa University School of Medicine
Tokyo
September 2006

Contents

Contributors

Amikura, Y., Department of Plastic and Reconstructive Surgery, Showa University School of Medicine, 1-5-8 Hatanodai, Shinagawa-ku, Tokyo 142-8666, Japan

Aoki, T., Department of Surgery, Division of Gastro-Intestinal Surgery, Showa University School of Medicine, 1-5-8 Hatanodai, Shinagawa-ku, Tokyo 142-8666, Japan

Aruga, T., Department of Emergency and Critical Care Medicine, Showa University School of Medicine, 1-5-8 Hatanodai, Shinagawa-ku, Tokyo 142-8555, Japan

Dohi, K., Department of Anatomy and Emergency and Critical Care Medicine, Showa University School of Medicine, 1-5-8 Hatanodai, Shinagawa-ku, Tokyo 142-8555, Japan

Ellis, E., Department of Pathology, University of Pittsburgh, 200 Lothrop St, 450 BST Pittsburgh, Pennsylvania, 15261 USA

Enami, Y., Department of Surgery, Division of Gastro-Intestinal Surgery, Showa University School of Medicine, 1-5-8 Hatanodai, Shinagawa-ku, Tokyo 142-8666, Japan

Geshi, E., Third Department of Internal Medicine, Showa University School of Medicine, 1-5-8 Hatanodai, Shinagawa-ku, Tokyo 142-8555, Japan

Hayashi, K., Department of Surgery, Division of Gastro-Intestinal Surgery, Showa University School of Medicine, 1-5-8 Hatanodai, Shinagawa-ku, Tokyo 142-8666, Japan

Honda, E., Department of Plastic and Reconstructive Surgery, Showa University School of Medicine, 1-5-8 Hatanodai, Shinagawa-ku, Tokyo 142-8666, Japan

Hosaka, Y., Department of Plastic and Reconstructive Surgery, Showa University School of Medicine, 1-5-8 Hatanodai, Shinagawa-ku, Tokyo 142-8666, Japan

Iso, Y., Third Department of Internal Medicine, Showa University School of Medicine, 1-5-8 Hatanodai, Shinagawa-ku, Tokyo 142-8555, Japan

Izumida, Y., Department of Surgery, Division of Gastro-Intestinal Surgery, Showa University School of Medicine, 1-5-8 Hatanodai, Shinagawa-ku, Tokyo 142-8666, Japan

Kamijo, R., Department of Biochemistry, School of Dentistry, Showa University, 1-5-8 Hatanodai, Shinagawa-ku, Tokyo 142-8555, Japan

Kao, B., Department of Plastic and Reconstructive Surgery, Showa University School of Medicine, 1-5-8 Hatanodai, Shinagawa-ku, Tokyo 142-8666, Japan

Katagiri, T., Third Department of Internal Medicine, Showa University School of Medicine, 1-5-8 Hatanodai, Shinagawa-ku, Tokyo 142-8555, Japan; Division of Pathophysiology, Research Center for Genomic Medicine, Saitama Medical School, 1397-1 Yamane, Hidaka, Saitama 350-1241, Japan

Kawachi, K., Division of Cardiology, Department of Internal Medicine, Showa University Fujigaoka Hospital, 1-30 Fujigaoka, Aoba-ku, Yokohama, Kanagawa 227-8501, Japan

Kikuyama, S., Department of Biology, School of Education, Waseda University, 1-6-1 Nishi-Waseda, Shinjuku-ku, Tokyo 169-8050, Japan

Koba, S., Third Department of Internal Medicine, Showa University School of Medicine, 1-5-8 Hatanodai, Shinagawa-ku, Tokyo 142-8555, Japan

Koike, T., Department of Orthopaedic Surgery, Osaka City University Medical School, 1-4-3 Asahimachi, Abeno-ku, Osaka 545-8585, Japan

Kudo, Y., Department of Orthopedic Surgery, Showa University School of Medicine, 1-5-8 Hatanodai, Shinagawa-ku, Tokyo 142-8555, Japan

Kusano, M., Department of Surgery, Division of Gastro-Intestinal Surgery, Showa University School of Medicine, 1-5-8 Hatanodai, Shinagawa-ku, Tokyo 142-8666, Japan

Kusano, T., Department of Surgery, Division of Gastro-Intestinal Surgery, Showa University School of Medicine, 1-5-8 Hatanodai, Shinagawa-ku, Tokyo 142-8666, Japan

Kusuyama, T., Third Department of Internal Medicine, Showa University School of Medicine, 1-5-8 Hatanodai, Shinagawa-ku, Tokyo 142-8666, Japan

Matsunaga, M., Gene Trophology Research Institute, Tokyo 130-0012, Japan

Matsuno, R., Department of Anatomy, Showa University School of Medicine, 1-5-8 Hatanodai, Shinagawa-ku, Tokyo 142-8555, Japan

Miki, T., Department of Pathology, University of Pittsburgh, 200 Lothrop St, 450 BST Pittsburgh, Pennsylvania, 15261 USA

Mitamura, K., Department of Pathology, University of Pittsburgh, 200 Lothrop St, 450 BST Pittsburgh, Pennsylvania, 15261 USA

Murai, N., Department of Surgery, Division of Gastro-Intestinal Surgery, Showa University School of Medicine, 1-5-8 Hatanodai, Shinagawa-ku, Tokyo 142-8666, Japan

Nakajo, S., Laboratory of Biochemistry, Yokohama College of Pharmacy, 601 Matano-cho, Yokohama, Kanagawa 245-0066, Japan

Nakamachi, T., Department of Anatomy, Showa University School of Medicine, 1-5-8 Hatanodai, Shinagawa-ku, Tokyo 142-8555, Japan

Nakaya, K., Faculty of Applied Life Sciences, Niigata University of Pharmacy and Applied Life Sciences, Niigata 956-8603, Japan

Niiya, T., Department of Surgery, Division of Gastro-Intestinal Surgery, Showa University School of Medicine, 1-5-8 Hatanodai, Shinagawa-ku, Tokyo 142-8666, Japan

Odaira, T., Department of Surgery, Division of Gastro-Intestinal Surgery, Showa University School of Medicine, 1-5-8 Hatanodai, Shinagawa-ku, Tokyo 142-8666, Japan

Ohba, M., Institute of Molecular Oncology, Showa University, 1-5-8 Hatanodai, Shinagawa-ku, Tokyo 142-8555, Japan

Ohbayashi, M., Department of Clinical Pharmacy, Showa University, 1-5-8 Hatanodai, Shinagawa-ku, Tokyo 142-8555, Japan

Ohno, F., Laboratory of Biological Chemistry, School of Pharmaceutical Sciences, Showa University, 1-5-8 Hatanodai, Shinagawa-ku, Tokyo 142-8555, Japan

Ohtaki, H., Department of Anatomy, Showa University School of Medicine, 1-5-8 Hatanodai, Shinagawa-ku, Tokyo 142-8555, Japan

Omori, Y., Third Department of Internal Medicine, Showa University School of Medicine, 1-5-8 Hatanodai, Shinagawa-ku, Tokyo 142-8555, Japan

Sakaida, I., Department of Gastroenterology & Hepatology, Yamaguchi University, Graduate School of Medicine, Minami Kogushi 1-1-1, Ube, Yamaguchi 755-8505, Japan

Sato, T., Third Department of Internal Medicine, Showa University School of Medicine, 1-5-8 Hatanodai, Shinagawa-ku, Tokyo 142-8555, Japan

Seki, T., Department of Anatomy II, Juntendo University School of Medicine, 2-1-1 Hongo, Bunkyo-ku, Tokyo 113-8421, Japan

Shimizu, S., Department of Pathophysiology, School of Pharmaceutical Sciences, Showa University, 1-5-8 Hatanodai, Shinagawa-ku, Tokyo 142-8555, Japan

Shimizu, Y., Department of Surgery, Division of Gastro-Intestinal Surgery, Showa University School of Medicine, 1-5-8 Hatanodai, Shinagawa-ku, Tokyo 142-8666, Japan

Shioda, S., Department of Anatomy, Showa University School of Medicine, 1-5-8 Hatanodai, Shinagawa-ku, Tokyo 142-8555, Japan

Shoji, M., Third Department of Internal Medicine, Showa University School of Medicine, 1-5-8 Hatanodai, Shinagawa-ku, Tokyo 142-8555, Japan

Soda, T., Third Department of Internal Medicine, Showa University School of Medicine, 1-5-8 Hatanodai, Shinagawa-ku, Tokyo 142-8555, Japan

Spees, J.L., Department of Medicine, Cardiovascular Research Institute, Stem Cell Core, University of Vermont, 208 South Park Drive, Suite 2, Colchester, VT, 05446 USA

Strom, S., Department of Pathology, University of Pittsburgh, 200 Lothrop St, 450 BST Pittsburgh, Pennsylvania, 15261 USA

Suzuki, H., Third Department of Internal Medicine, Showa University School of Medicine, 1-5-8 Hatanodai, Shinagawa-ku, Tokyo 142-8555, Japan

Takada, T., Department of Periodontology, School of Dentistry, Showa University, 1-5-8 Hatanodai, Shinagawa-ku, Tokyo 142-8555, Japan

Takaoka, K., Department of Orthopaedic Surgery, Osaka City University Medical School, 1-4-3 Asahimachi, Abeno-ku, Osaka 545-8585, Japan

Takeyama, Y., Division of Cardiology, Department of Internal Medicine, Showa University Fujigaoka Hospital, 1-30 Fujigaoka, Aoba-ku, Yokohama, Kanagawa 227-8501, Japan

Tomizuka, Y., Department of Plastic and Reconstructive Surgery, Showa University School of Medicine, 1-5-8 Hatanodai, Shinagawa-ku, Tokyo 142-8666, Japan

Tomotake, K., Department of Surgery, Division of Gastro-Intestinal Surgery, Showa University School of Medicine, 1-5-8 Hatanodai, Shinagawa-ku, Tokyo 142-8666, Japan

Tomoyasu, S., Department of Hematology, Showa University School of Medicine, 1-5-8 Hatanodai, Shinagawa-ku, Tokyo 142-8555, Japan

XVIII

Toyoda, H., Department of Orthopaedic Surgery, Osaka City University Medical School, 1-4-3 Asahimachi, Abeno-ku, Osaka 545-8585, Japan

Tsunoda, F., Third Department of Internal Medicine, Showa University School of Medicine, 1-5-8 Hatanodai, Shinagawa-ku, Tokyo 142-8555, Japan

Wakabayashi, K., Division of Cardiology, Department of Internal Medicine, Showa University Fujigaoka Hospital, 1-30 Fujigaoka, Aoba-ku, Yokohama, Kanagawa 227-8501, Japan

Watanabe, J., Department of Anatomy, Showa University School of Medicine, 1-5-8 Hatanodai, Shinagawa-ku, Tokyo 142-8555, Japan; Department of Biology, School of Education, Waseda University, 1-6-1 Nishi-Waseda, Shinjuku-ku, Tokyo 169-8050, Japan

Yamada, K., Department of Surgery, Division of Gastro-Intestinal Surgery, Showa University School of Medicine, 1-5-8 Hatanodai, Shinagawa-ku, Tokyo 142-8666, Japan

Yamamoto, T., Department of Clinical Pharmacy, Showa University, 1-5-8 Hatanodai, Shinagawa-ku, Tokyo 142-8555, Japan

Yasuda, D., Department of Surgery, Division of Gastro-Intestinal Surgery, Showa University School of Medicine, 1-5-8 Hatanodai, Shinagawa-ku, Tokyo 142-8666, Japan

Yasuda, M., Department of Clinical Pharmacy, Showa University, 1-5-8 Hatanodai, Shinagawa-ku, Tokyo 142-8555, Japan

Yofu, S., Department of Anatomy, Showa University School of Medicine, 1-5-8 Hatanodai, Shinagawa-ku, Tokyo 142-8555, Japan; Gene Trophology Research Institute, Tokyo 130-0012, Japan

Yokota, Y., Third Department of Internal Medicine, Showa University School of Medicine, 1-5-8 Hatanodai, Shinagawa-ku, Tokyo 142-8555, Japan

Zhao, B., Department of Biochemistry, School of Dentistry, Showa University, 1-5-8 Hatanodai, Shinagawa-ku, Tokyo 142-8555, Japan

Color Plates

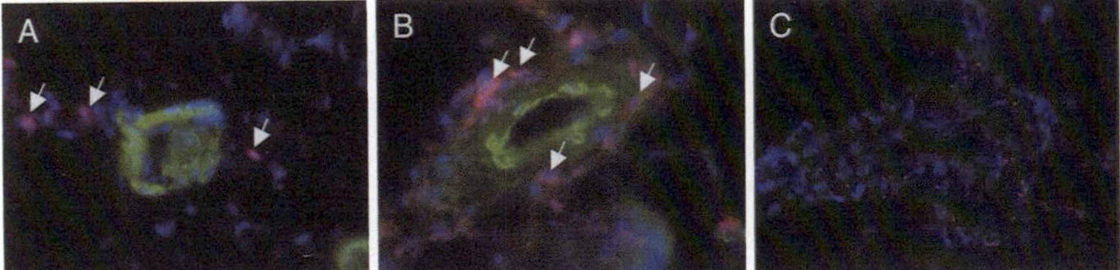

Bone marrow progenitor cells participate in repair/remodeling during monocrota-line-induced pulmonary hypertension. A) Lung section from a control rat that received BMT but no MCT (6 weeks after BMT). Green (ALEXA 488): α-SMA staining of a blood vessel. Red (ALEXA 594): antibody staining of GFP-positive bone marrowderived cells. B) GFP-positive bone marrow cells (red) surround a blood vessel of a MCT-treated chimeric rat (6 weeks after BMT, 3 weeks after MCT). C) Y chromosome in situ hybridization (pink dots) to confirm the engraft-ment of male bone marrow-derived cells in the female host. Blue nuclei are stained with DAPI. Please refer also to the color plate in the front of this book. (p 50)

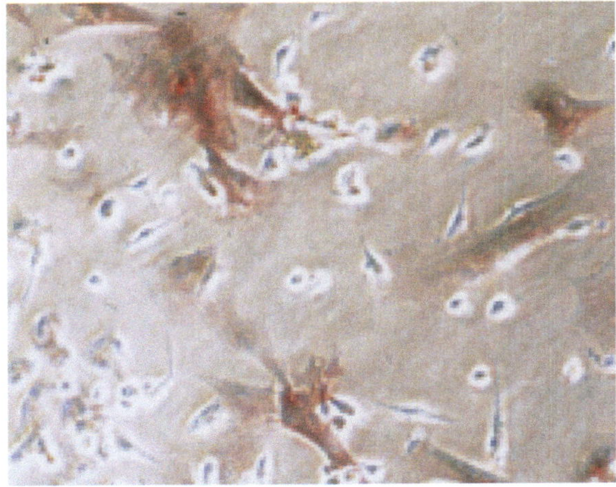

Contribution of bone marrow-derived cells to neointimal formation. Bone marrow cells differentiated into smooth muscle-like cells, which expressed α-SMA. (8 days after cell culture). (p 72)

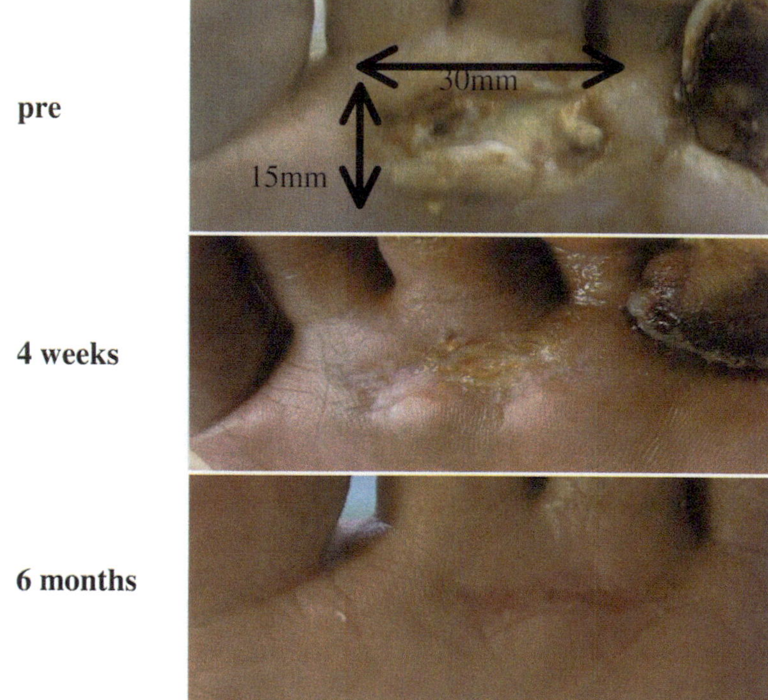

Ulcer healing process. Macroscopic findings; intractable ulcer sized 30 mm × 15 mm healed within 4 weeks. And after 6 months, ulcer scar also disappeared. (p 99)

Part I
Digestive and Integumentary System

Hepatocyte transplantation for liver disease

Keitaro Mitamura, Ewa Ellis, Toshio Miki, Stephen Strom

Department of Pathology, University of Pittsburgh, 200 Lothrop St, 450 BST Pittsburgh, Pennsylvania 15261, USA

Summary. There is a need for new therapies for support of liver function. Hepatocyte transplantation (Htx) has been used to support liver function in acute or chronic liver disease and as a "cellular therapy" for metabolic liver disease. Transplants in human patients mirror the results of animal studies and indicate that Htx increases survival of acute liver failure patients and partially or completely corrects metabolic liver disease. These promising results suggest that Htx could be an inexpensive and effective treatment for liver disease. Clinical programs are now established in at least 13 different centers in 9 different countries.

Key words. Hepatocyte transplantation, metabolic liver disease, acute liver failure

1 Introduction

The number of patients on the waiting list for whole organ transplantation (Oltx) continues to increase while in any given year less than 1/3 of the patients will receive a transplant. Although still experimental, HTx has some theoretical advantages over liver transplantation. The benefits of cell transplants include the ease in timing of the transplants, a less invasive and less costly procedure and cell transplants proven to have fewer and less serious complications than OLTx.

Preclinical studies indicate that transplanted hepatocytes retain normal hepatic function, survive for the life-time of the recipient (8, 13–15, 20–21) and can significantly improve or correct prothrombin time (PT), serum albumin, bilirubin levels, hepatic encephalopathy and survival in end-stage

4

cirrhosis (1, 3, 7, 17, 28). Metabolic defects in bilirubin metabolism, albumin secretion, copper excretion, familial intrahepatic cholestasis and tyrosinemia have been corrected by HTx (7, 10) (19, 27 and 28 for reviews).

2 Hepatocyte transplantation for acute liver failure and chronic liver disease

Hepatocyte transplantation has been an effective therapy for acute liver failure and end-stage liver disease associated with cirrhosis (1, 3, 7, 17, 19, 27–28). Promising preclinical results lead to attempts to support patients with acute or chronic liver failure by HTx. In a series of 22 patients awaiting liver transplantation, HTx was performed to provide liver function. There were 11 survivors and 7 deaths in this group. Four patients not receiving a cell transplant were included as controls. The treatment group showed over 60% survival while there were no survivors in the control group (19, 25–28). These initial studies suggest that those patients receiving HTx have a survival advantage as compared to those who do not.

3 Hepatocyte transplantation to support liver function and facilitate regeneration of the native liver

While most of the liver failure patients described above received Oltx following the hepatocyte transplant, two of the patients recovered from acute liver failure following cell transplantation without having to receive the OLTx (5, reviewed in 27, 28). In both cases the improvement was sufficiently rapid that the patients were subsequently removed from the transplant list. Full recovery, took additional weeks. Results with these 2 patients agrees well with that of Soriano et al.,(22) who reported the complete recovery of pediatric patient with hepatic failure fcllowing HTx. It is believed that HTx kept the patient alive, providing time for the native liver to regenerate. These reports indicate that HTx can be an effective treatment for fulminant hepatic failure.

4 Cellular therapy of metabolic liver disease

Several animal models of liver disease have been discovered or created. Many have been used to test the hypothesis that cell transplantation alone could correct the clinical symptoms of the disease and corrections of these diseases were attained by Htx. Reports indicate that partial or complete corrections of Crigler-Najjar, Factor 7 or Ornithine Transcarbamylase (OTC) or argininosuccinate lyase deficiency, Glycogen Storage or infantile Refsum disease, was attained in patients following Htx (4, 6, 9, 16, 23–24, 27–28). These studies support the idea that Htx can provide correction of genetic defects in liver function.

5 Hepatocyte transplantation challenges and future directions

The most significant obstacle to expanding hepatocyte therapy of liver disease is the shortage of useful hepatocytes for the transplant procedure (18). Future studies will likely examine the use of xenotransplants, immortalized cells and stem cell derived hepatocytes (2, 11–12, 17, 29). If suitable cell sources can be identified, an extensive and rigorous investigation of the full potential of hepatocyte transplants can be conducted. Transplant and immunosuppression protocols will need to be standardized by the participating laboratories. The close ties and cooperation that has developed between investigators at the different transplant centers will insure that technology will be improved and shared with relative ease.

References

1. Ahmad, T. A., S. Eguchi, K. Yanaga, S. Miyamoto, Y. Kamohara, H. Fujioka, J. Furui, and T. Kanematsu. 2002. Role of intrasplenic hepatocyte transplantation in improving survival and liver regeneration after hepatic resection in cirrhotic rats. Cell Transplant 11:399–402.
2. Avital, I., C. Feraresso, T. Aoki, T. Hui, J. Rozga, A. Demetriou, and M. Muraca. 2002. Bone marrow-derived liver stem cell and mature hepatocyte engraftment in livers undergoing rejection. Surgery 132:384–90.
3. Cai, J., M. Ito, H. Nagata, K. A. Westerman, D. Lafleur, J. R. Chowdhury, P. Leboulch, and I. J. Fox. 2002. Treatment of liver failure in rats with end-stage cirrhosis by transplantation of immortalized hepatocytes. Hepatology 36: 386–94.
4. Dhawan, A., R. R. Mitry, R. D. Hughes, S. Lehec, C. Terry, S. Bansal, R. Arya, J. J. Wade, A. Verma, N. D. Heaton, M. Rela, and G. Mieli-Vergani. 2004. Hepatocyte transplantation for inherited factor VII deficiency. Transplantation 78:1812–4.
5. Fisher, R. A., D. Bu, M. Thompson, J. Tisnado, U. Prasad, R. Sterling, M. Posner, and S. Strom. 2000. Defining hepatocellular chimerism in a liver failure patient bridged with hepatocyte infusion. Transplantation 69:303–7.
6. Fox, I. J., J. R. Chowdhury, S. S. Kaufman, T. C. Goertzen, N. R. Chowdhury, P. I. Warkentin, K. Dorko, B. V. Sauter, and S. C. Strom. 1998. Treatment of

the Crigler-Najjar syndrome type I with hepatocyte transplantation. N Engl J Med 338:1422–6.

7. Fox, I. J., and J. Roy-Chowdhury. 2004. Hepatocyte transplantation. J Hepatol 40:878–86.

8. Gupta, S., E. Aragona, R. P. Vemuru, K. K. Bhargava, R. D. Burk, and J. R. Chowdhury. 1991. Permanent engraftment and function of hepatocytes delivered to the liver: implications for gene therapy and liver repopulation. Hepatology 14:144–9.

9. Horslen, S. P., T. C. McCowan, T. C. Goertzen, P. I. Warkentin, H. B. Cai, S. C. Strom, and I. J. Fox. 2003. Isolated hepatocyte transplantation in an infant with a severe urea cycle disorder. Pediatrics 111:1262–7.

10. Irani, A. N., H. Malhi, S. Slehria, G. R. Gorla, I. Volenberg, M. L. Schilsky, and S. Gupta. 2001. Correction of liver disease following transplantation of normal rat hepatocytes into Long-Evans Cinnamon rats modeling Wilson's disease. Mol Ther 3:302–9.

11. Kobayashi, N., T. Fujiwara, K. A. Westerman, Y. Inoue, M. Sakaguchi, H. Noguchi, M. Miyazaki, J. Cai, N. Tanaka, I. J. Fox, and P. Leboulch. 2000. Prevention of acute liver failure in rats with reversibly immortalized human hepatocytes. Scence 287:1258–62.

12. Miki, T., T. Lehmann, H. Cai, D. B. Stoltz, and S. C. Strom. 2005. Stem cell characteristics of amniotic epithelial cells. Stem Cells 23:1549–59, 2005.

13. Mito, M., H. Ebata, M. Kusano, T. Onishi, T. Saito, and S. Sakamoto. 1979. Morphology and function of isolated hepatocytes transplanted into rat spleen. Transpl 28:499–505.

14. Mito, M., M. Kusano, and Y. Kawaura. 1992. Hepatocyte transplantation in man. Transplant Proc 24:3052–3.

15. Mito, M., M. Kusano, and Sawa, M. 1993. Hepatocyte transplantation for hepatic failure. Transplant Rev 7:35.

16. Muraca, M., G. Gerunda, D. Neri, M. T. Vilei, A. Granato, P. Feltracco, M. Meroni, G. Giron, and A. B. Burlina. 2002. Hepatocyte transplantation as a treatment for glycogen storage disease type Ia. Lancet 359:317–8.

17. Nagata, H., M. Ito, J. Cai, A. S. Edge, J. L. Platt, and I. J. Fox. 2003. Treatment of cirrhosis and liver failure in rats by hepatocyte xenotransplantation. Gastroenterology 124:422–31.

18. Nakazawa, F., H. Cai, T. Miki, K. Dorko, A. Abdelmeguid, J. Walldorf, T. Lehmann, and S. Strom. 2002. Human hepatocyte isolation from cadaver donor liver, p. 147–158, Proceedings of Falk Symposium, Hepatocyte Transplantation, vol. 126. Kouwer Academic Publishers, Lancaster, UK.

19. Ohashi, K., F. Park, and M. A. Kay. 2001. Hepatocyte transplantation: clinical and experimental application. J Mol Med 79:617–30.

20. Overturf, K., M. Al-Dhalimy, R. Tanguay, M. Brantly, C. N. Ou, M. Finegold, and M. Grompe. 1996. Hepatocytes corrected by gene therapy are selected in vivo in a murine model of hereditary tyrosinaemia type I. Nat Genet 12:266–73.

21. Ponder, K. P., S. Gupta, F. Leland, G. Darlington, M. Finegold, J. DeMayo, F. D. Ledley, J. R. Chowdhury, and S. L. Woo. 1991. Mouse hepatocytes

migrate to liver parenchyma and function indefinitely after intrasplenic transplantation. Proc Natl Acad Sci U S A 88:1217–21.
22. Soriano, H. E. 2002. Liver cell transplantation: human applications in adults and children, p. 99–115, Proceedings of Falk Symposium, Hepatocyte Transplantation, vol. 126. Kouwer Academic Publishers, Lancaster, UK.
23. Stephenne, X., M. Najimi, F. Smets, R. Reding, J. Goyet, and E. M. Sokal, Cryopreserved liver cell transplantation controls OTC deficient patient while awaiting liver transplantation. Am J Transpl 2058–2061, 2005.
24. Stephenne, X., M. Najimi, C. Sibille, M-C. Nassogne, F. Smets, and E. M. Sokal, Sustained engraftment ant tissue enzyme activity after liver cell transplantation for arginosuccinate lyase deficiency. Gastroenterology 1317–1323, 2006.
25. Strom, S. C., R. A. Fisher, M. T. Thompson, A. J. Sanyal, P. E. Cole, J. M. Ham, and M. P. Posner. 1997. Hepatocyte transplantation as a bridge to orthotopic liver transplantation in terminal liver failure. Transplantation 63:559–69.
26. Strom, S. C., R. A. Fisher, W. S. Rubinstein, J. A. Barranger, R. B. Towbin, M. Charron, L. Mieles, L. A. Pisarov, K. Dorko, M. T. Thompson, and J. Reyes. 1997. Transplantation of human hepatocytes. Transplant Proc 29:2103–6.
27. Strom, S. C., J. R. Chowdhury, and I. J. Fox. 1999. Hepatocyte transplantation for the treatment of human disease. Semin Liver Dis 19:39–48.
28. Strom S. P. Bruzzoni, H. Cai, E. Ellis, T. Lehmann, K. Mitamura, and T. Miki, (2006) Human hepatocyte transplantation, clinical experience. Cell Transplantation 15 (suppl) S105–S110.
29. Wege, H., H. T. Le, M. S. Chui, L. Liu, J. Wu, R. Giri, H. Malhi, B. S. Sappal, V. Kumaran, S. Gupta, and M. A. Zern. 2003. Telomerase reconstitution immortalizes human fetal hepatocytes without disrupting their differentiation potential. Gastroenterology 124:432–44.

Liver regeneration with the resolution of fibrosis by bone marrow cell infusion therapy

Isao Sakaida

Department of Gastroenterology & Hepatology, Yamaguchi University, Graduate School of Medicine Minami Kogushi 1-1-1, Ube, Yamaguchi 755-8505, Japan

Summary. Infused (transplanted) green fluorescent protein (GFP)-positive bone marrow cells (BMCs) migrated into the peri-portal regions of the cirrhotic mouse liver induced continuous CCl_4 injection without irradiation (without bone marrow ablation). The infused GFP-positive BMCs differentiated into hepatoblasts detected with Liv2-antibody and then differentiated into albumin-producing hepatocytes. The differentiation "niche" induced by persistent liver damage due to continuous CCl_4 injection seems to be an essential factor. Microarry analysis showed that at an early stage after BMC infusion through mouse tail vein, the genes related to degradation of extracellular matrix (ECM) e.g. MMP-9 were activated. BMC infusion improved liver fibrosis and the survival rate. Recent our finding indicates that mesencymal bone marrow cells will differentiate to hepatocytes and FGF2 will accelerate this differentiation of BMC to hepatocyte. Based on the results obtained in basic research using the GFP/CCl_4 model, human trials are now undergoing.

Key words. Bone marrow cell, stem cell, fibrosis, regeneration, matrix metalloproteinase

1 Introduction

Liver transplantation is one of the most effective therapies to cure the patients with advanced liver diseases e.g. liver cirrhosis. However, transplantation has many problems such as a lack of donor, operative damage, rejection and high expense. Cell transplantation (infusion) therapy should be a minimally invasive procedure with fewer potential complications.

Regenerative medicine using stem cells is an attractive treatment for patients with severe liver disease. The capacity of bone marrow cells (BMCs) to differentiate into hepatocytes and intestinal cells was confirmed through the detection of the Y chromosome in an autopsy analysis of human female recipients of BMCs from male donors (Alison MR et al. 2000, Korbling M et al. 2000, Okamoto R et al. 2002, Theise ND et al. 2000). We developed a new in vivo model named the "Green Fluorescent Protein (GFP) / carbon tetrachloride (CCl_4) model" (Terai S et al. 2003), used to monitor the differentiation of BMCs into functional hepatocytes. The newest findings from the GFP/CCl_4 model have been described and discussed in this manuscript compared to recent other findings.

2 Bone marrow cells for the source of liver regeneration

If we limit the definition of stem cells to their ability to self renew and reconstitute a given tissue in vivo, hepatocytes fulfill both criteria. However, hepatocyte transplantation has very rarely produced therapeutic effects in human clinical trials, mainly because their numbers are too low to achieve a biological effect (Fox IJ et al. 1998, Muraca M et al. 2002). Under certain conditions, when hepatocyte replication is blocked, bipotent oval cells profilerate and participate in liver regeneration. However, the fact that they have been shown to generate hepatocellular carcinoma and cholangiocarcinoma cells in rodents is a concern for their use for cell therapy.

As a result, bone marrow cells are now being considered. The capacity of bone marrow cells (BMCs) to differentiate into hepatocytes was found using Y chromosome detection in an autopsy analysis of human female recipients of BMCs from male donors as described previously (Alison MR et al. 2000, Theise ND et al. 2000). BMC transplantation itself is an established treatment for hematological diseases. These results suggest that bone marrow is an attractive cell source for regenerative medicine, because obtaining BMCs is easier than other tissue specific stem cells. In the field of cardiovascular diseases, clinical studies have been performed to evaluate the use of BMCs in regenerating the myocardium and vessels of limb ischemia (Kobayashi Y et al. 2002, Stamm C et al. 2003, Tateishi-Yuyama E et al. 2003, Wexler SA et al. 2003). Although various theories explain the existence of pluripotent stem cells in BMCs, the exact composition of stem cells among BMCs remains unclear. The following cell types are known to exist in bone marrow: hematopoietic stem cells (HSC) (Krause DS et al. 2001, Lagasse E et al. 2000), side population cells (SP) (Uchida N et al. 2001) and mesenchymal stem cells (MSC) (Pittenger MF et al. 1999). Although past studies used the existing antibodies and techniques, there have been no studies based on the findings associated with natural liver development.

Hematopoietic stem cells (HSCs) have been shown to adopt the phenotype of the recipient cells with fusion (Terada N et al. 2002, Ying QL et al. 2002). This fusion event has been demonstrated to occur between resident hepatocytes and myelomonocytes (Camargo FD et al. 2004, Willenbring H et al. 2004), and also in normal mice using the Cre-cox system (Alvarez-Dolado M et al. 2003).

However, using the same approach, Harris et al. recently demonstrated that epithelial cells can develop from bone marrow cells without cell fusion (Harris RG et al. 2004). Also, recent publications have suggested that bone marrow-derived hepatocytes may originate from the mesenchymal compartment, rather than the hematopoietic compartment (Lee KD et al. 2004, Jiang Y et al. 2002).

3 Bone marrow cell infusion model with chronic liver injury (The GFP/CCl4 model)

To investigate whether BMCs will be able to be used to repair liver damage, the GFP/CCl$_4$ model has been developed (Terai S et al. 2003). In this model (Fig. 1), 0.5 ml/kg of carbon tetrachloride (CCl$_4$) is administered twice weekly to C57BL/6 female mice to induce liver cirrhosis, and then green fluorescent protein (GFP)-positive BMCs obtained from GFP-Tg mice (C57BL6/ Tg14 (act-EGFP) OsbY01 mice) (Okabe M et al. 1997) are infused through the tail vein without the irradiation of bone marrow ablation (donor and recipient mice are of the same strain). In this model, 1×10^5 GFP-positive BMCs were infused without culture. By analyzing the GFP-positive BMCs in the recipient mice, the repopulation and differentiation of BMCs under continuous liver injury were evaluated. Immunostaining using anti-GFP antibodies (Shinoda K et al. 1992) showed that GFP-positive BMCs migrated into the marginal area of the hepatic lobule starting one day after BMC infusion, and with time, the distribution of GFP-positive BMCs expanded while forming a hepatic cord towards the central vein. The use of Liv2, a hepatoblast-specific antibody (Watanabe T et al. 2002) also showed that BMCs first differentiate into Liv2-positive hepatoblasts and then differentiate into albumin-positive hepatocytes. Furthermore, the level of serum albumin significantly increases with time in recipient mice. These findings suggest that the GFP/CCl$_4$ model can be used to understand the process of differentiation of BMC into hepatocytes. On the other hand, GFP-positive cells were not detected in the liver tissue of control mice (no damage) following BMC infusion. Persistent liver damage induced by CCl$_4$

GFP/CCl4 model

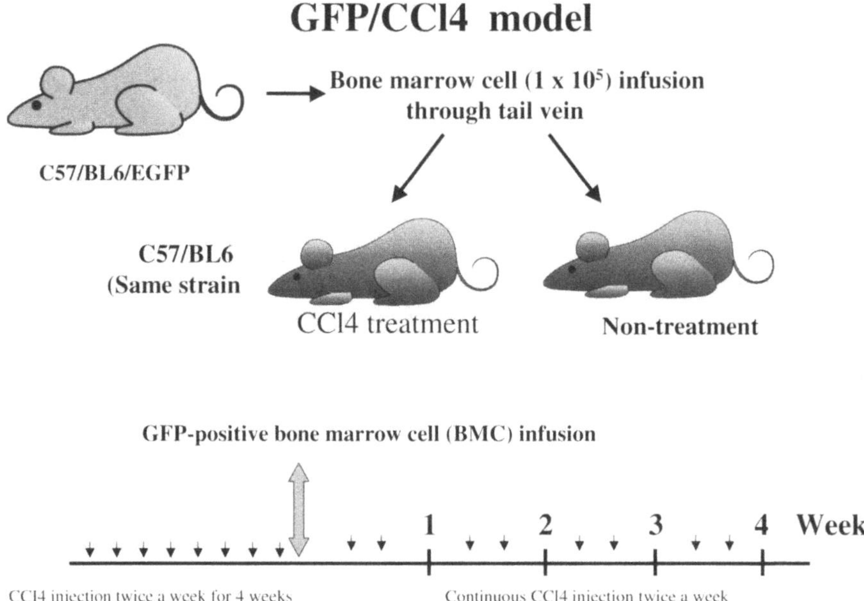

Fig. 1. Experimental protocol for the GFP/CCl$_4$ model.

injection is important for producing a specific differentiation "niche" in order to activate the plasticity of BMCs and their subsequent differentiation into hepatocytes. Oval cells were thought to be one of the types of hepatic stem cells derived from the Canal of Hering following severe liver damage (Grisham JW et al. 1997, Petersen BE et al. 1998). Based on the findings of Petersen et al. that under some conditions, oval cells are derived from bone marrow cells (Petersen BE et al. 1999), we also analyzed the activation of oval cells using a specific oval cell marker, A6 antibody. A6-positive cells were detected at the peri-portal region one week after BMC transplantation in the GFP/CCl$_4$ model, but A6-positive oval cells did not increase in the four weeks after BMC infusion in the GFP/CCl$_4$ model. We could not detect A6-positive cells that also express GFP in the liver after BMC infusion. These results suggest that some signals that activate oval cells are induced by BMC infusion into CCl$_4$-induced cirrhotic livers, but that oval cells might not be derived from infused BMCs. BMCs infused into the GFP/CCl$_4$ model differentiated into hepatoblast phenotypes, then differentiated into albumin-producing hepatocytes in the "differentiation niche" created by persistent CCl$_4$ injection. On the other hand, the contribution to parenchymal regeneration from bone marrow was minor and oval cells/small hepatocyte like progenitor cells contributed after liver cell injury when the bone marrow ablation was performed (Vig P et al. 2006). Whether the bone marrow ablation was performed or not may explain these different findings. In our model, we infused (transplanted) bone marrow cells without bone marrow ablation resulting in the contribution of liver regeneration with the resolution of liver fibrosis.

4 Effect of BMC infusion

Infused BMCs differentiated into albumin-producing hepatocytes, leading to an increase in the serum albumin level. Interestingly, an improvement in liver fibrosis after BMC infusion was seen (Sakaida I et al. 2004). Although the exact mechanism of fibrolysis remains unclear, infused BMCs migrate along with the fibers with the strong expression of matrix metalloproteinase (MMP)-9, resulting in the resolution of fibrosis (Figs. 2, 3, 4). The degradation of the extracellular matrix presumably leads to improved liver function resulting in better survival in mice following BMC infusion. To clarify which fraction of BMCs is responsible for this improvement of liver function and resolution of liver fibrosis, Liv8 antibody was developed (Yamamoto N

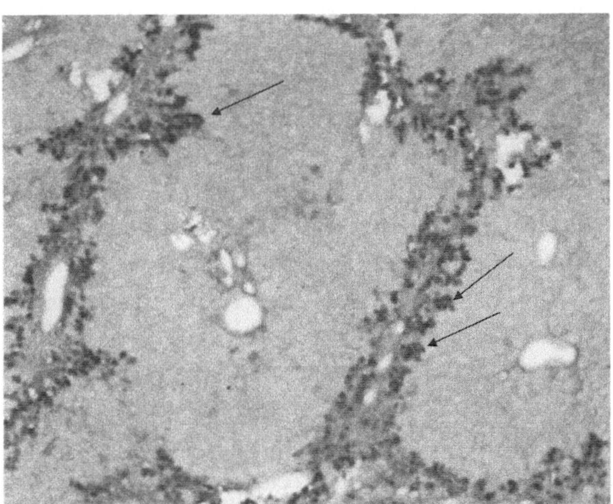

Fig. 2. GFP and Sirius red staining. Migrated bone marrow cells (arrows) are seen along with the fibers.

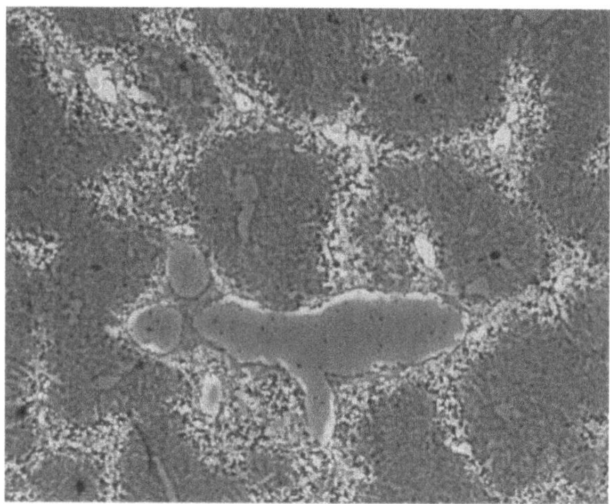

Fig. 3. In situ zymography. Migrated bone marrow cells are expressing MMP-9 and resolving the gelatin (extracellular matrix) leading to the resolution of liver fibrosis.

et al. 2004). The mouse fetal liver at 11.5 functions as a definitive hematopoietic organ and Liv8-positve cells of the fetal liver at E11.5 include c-kit-positive immature hematopoietic cells and CD-45 positive lymphoid cells. These results indicate that Liv8-positive BMCs include almost all immature and mature hematopoietic cells. We also analyzed differences in liver fibrosis following infusion of Liv8-positive or Liv8-negative BMCs. Our results showed that Liv8-negative BMC infusion improved liver function (e.g. serum albumin level) and fibrosis more than Liv8-positive BMC infusion. These results show that subpopulations of Liv-8 negative cells (non-hematopietic cells) will be useful for curing liver cirrhosis. Our double-fluorecence data may also indicate that infused BMCs seem to become stellate cells, in agreement with a recent report (Forbes SJ 2004), although the number was very small in our experimental model. Again whether bone marrow ablation was performed (transplantation) or not (cell infusion) may lead BMCs to different phenotypes. This result seems to be contradictory to our result for the resolution of liver fibrosis by BMC infusion, because differentiated stellate cells may produce collagens. Our preliminary results indicated a reduced mRNA expression of type I procollagen, TGF-β1, and no change of HGF mRNA expression in the liver one week after BMC infusion compared with the CCl4-alone treated liver. Migrated BMCs seemed to reduce the fine network pattern of activated stellate cells. Thus, infused BMCs may affect activated stellate cells to reduce their number; e.g. by

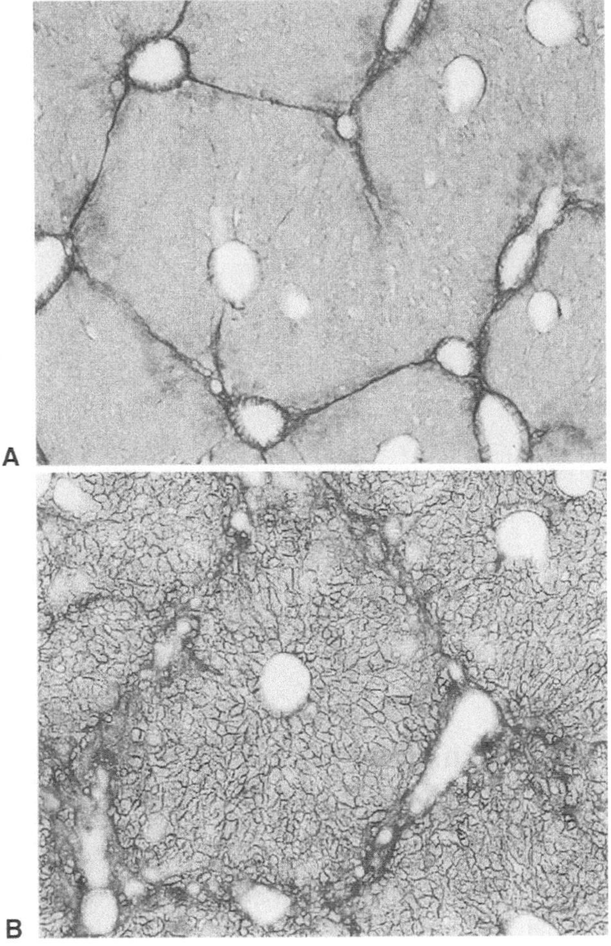

Fig. 4. Resolution of liver fibrosis after bone marrow cell infusion.
A: CCl4 treatment alone for 8 weeks.
B: CCl4 treatment with bone marrow cell infusion (4 weeks after infusion, total 8 weeks).

leading them to apoptosis. However, further examinations are necessary to determine the exact relationship between BMCs and resident stellate cells. BMC infusion into liver cirrhotic mice has two effects: BMC differentiation into albumin, producing hepatocytes with the resolution of liver fibrosis. These effects of BMC infusion accelerate the improvement of liver function and the survival rate (Fig. 5).

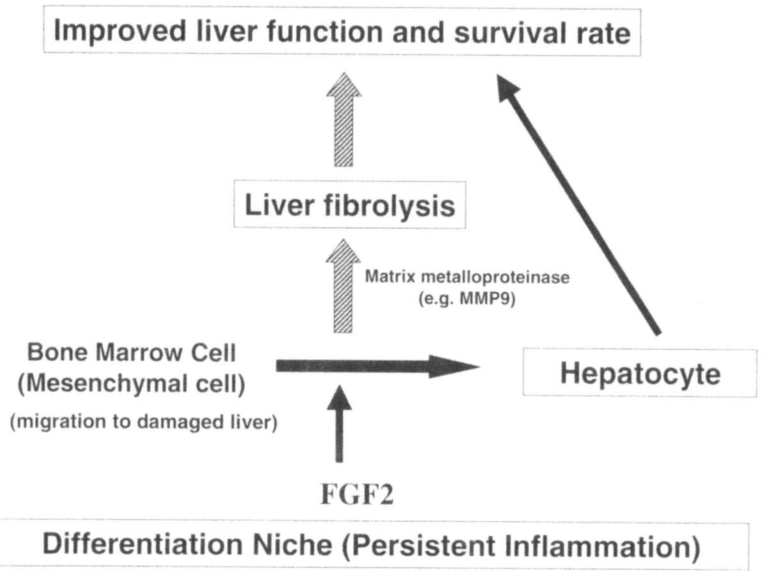

Fig. 5. Summary of GFP/CCl$_4$ model.

5 Molecular mechanisms of BMC differentiation

The differentiation of BMCs into hepatocytes in the fumarylacetoacetate hydrolase (FAH) model was thought to show the importance of cell fusion in the differentiation of HSC into hepatocytes (Wang X et al. 2003, Vassilopoulos G et al. 2003). However, other groups have reported little evidence of in vivo cell fusion during the differentiation of BMCs into other cell lineages (Lanus A et al. 2003). We analyzed the cell fusion rate using cultured Neo-resistant ES cells and GFP-positive BMCs under the same culture conditions as Terada N et al. (Terada N et al. 2002) (cell fusion rate of $1/10^5$–10^6) and found similar cell fusion rates in our in vitro assay. Mouse hepatocytes have ploidy values of 2N, 4N, 8N or 16N. Cell fusion of diploid (2N) BMCs with hepatocytes produces cells with ploidy values of 4N, 6N, 10N or 18N. It seems that the variety of ploidy values would make it very difficult to analyze cell fusion. We analyzed the DNA ploidy patterns of isolated primary hepatocytes in persistent CCl$_4$-damaged mice with and without BMC infusion at four weeks. We were able to isolate around 1.2×10^8 hepatocytes from recipient mice at four weeks using a two-step collagenase method and analyzed the DNA ploidy patterns with FACS. We found 2N, 4N, 8N and 16N DNA bands. Comparisons of these DNA ploidy patterns showed that the 2N and 4N band were similar, but the peak representing the 8N and 16N bands were slightly different. These results suggest that cell fusion could have occurred in the GFP/CCl$_4$ model but further examinations are necessary. Although we could not neglect the possibility that cell fusion had occurred in our model, BMC seemed to differentiate into Liv2 positive hepatoblasts and functional hepatocytes, mainly without cell fusion. Also, we analyzed the mechanism of this plasticity using DNA chips, which are recently developed tools of genetic analysis (Schena M et al. 1995). While it is possible to obtain vast amounts of genetic data using DNA chips, interpretation of the factors involved in gene expression requires the application of a statistical technique such as a self-organizing map (SOM) to visualize the vast amounts of complicated and multidimensional data (Xiao L et al. 2003). In this analysis, we made a specific equation to extract genes that regulate the differentiation of BMCs into hepatocytes. Genes related to morphology were dramatically activated at an early stage, while genes associated with hepatocyte differentiation were up-regulated at a later stage in the GFP/CCl$_4$ model. In the early stage after BMC infusion, we found that genes such as FGF and c-kit, as well as HOX and HLH transcription factors, might have been important. In later stages, genes associated with metabolic function, such as hepatocyte nuclear factor 4 (HNF4) and glucose-6-phosohatase (G6Pase) isomerase, were induced, suggesting that at four weeks after BMCs infusion, infused BMC began to assume some of the metabolic functions of hepatocytes (Omori K et al. 2004). Although many details remain unconfirmed, the Microarray-SOM analysis for the GFP/CCl$_4$ model confirmed the idea that BMCs differentiated into immature cells and then differentiated into mature hepatocytes. This information will be useful for understanding the mechanism of the plasticity of BMCs in the GFP/CCl$_4$ model. Recent finding indicates that fibroblast growth factor 2 (FGF2) will accelerate the differentiation of BMCs to hepatocytes with increased resolution of liver fibrosis and survival rate (Ishikawa et al. 2005).

Although there are many questions remaining to be clarified, cell therapy using BMCs is a promising candidate for new therapeutic modalities for advanced liver diseases.

References

Alison MR, Poulsom R, Jeffery R, Dhillon AP, Quaglia A, Jacob J, Novelli M, Prentice G, Williamson J, Wright NA. (2000) Hepatocytes from non-hepatic adult stem cells. Nature 406:257.

Alvarez-Dolado M, Pardal R, Garcia-Verdugo JM, Fike JR, Lee HO, Pfeffer K, Lois C, Morrison SJ, Alvarez-Buylla A. (2003) Fusion of bone-marrow-derived cells with Purkinje neurons, cardiomyocytes and hepatocytes. Nature 425:968–973.

Camargo FD, Finegold M, Goodell MA. (2004) Hematopoietic myelomonocytic cells are the major source of hepatocyte fusion partners. J Clin Invest 113:1266–1270.

Forbes SJ, Russo FP, Rey V, Burra P, Rugge M, Wright NA, Alison MR. (2004) A significant proportion of myofibroblasts are of bone marrow origin in human liver fibrosis. Gastroenterology 126:955–963.

Fox IJ, Chowdhury JR, Kaufman SS, Goertzen TC, Chowdhury NR, Warkentin PI, Dorko K, Sauter BV, Strom SC. (1998) Treatment of the Crigler-Najjar syndrome type I with hepatocyte transplantation. N Engl J Med 338:1422–1426.

Grisham JW, Thorgeirsson SS. (1997) Liver stem cells. Potten CS eds. Stem Cells. Academic Press London, pp 233–282.

Harris RG, Herzog EL, Bruscia EM, Grove JE, Van Arnam JS, Krause DS. (2004) Lack of a fusion requirement for development of bone marrow-derived epithelia. Science 305:90–93.

Ianus A, Holz GG, Theise ND, Hussain MA. (2003) In vivo derivation of glucose-competent pancreatic endocrine cells from bone marrow without evidence of cell fusion. J Clin Invest 111:843–850.

Ishikawa T, Terai S, Urata Y, Marumoto Y, Aoyama K, Sakaida I, Murata T, Nishina H, Shinoda K, Uchimura S, Hamamoto Y, Okita K. (2005) Fibroblast growth factor 2 facilitates the differentiation of transplanted bone marrow cells into hepatocytes. Cell Tissue Res. 14:1–11.

Jiang Y, Jahagirdar BN, Reinhardt RL, Schwartz RE, Keene CD, Ortiz-Gonzalez XR, Reyes M, Lenvik T, Lund T, Blackstad M, Du J, Aldrich S, Lisberg A, Low WC, Largaespada DA, Verfaillie CM. (2002) Pluripotency of mesenchymal stem cells derived from adult marrow. Nature 418:41–49.

Krause DS, Theise ND, Collector MI, Henegariu O, Hwang S, Gardner R, Neutzel S, Sharkis SJ. (2001) Multi-organ, multi-lineage engraftment by a single bone marrow-derived stem cell. Cell 105:369–377.

Kobayashi T, Hamano K, Li TS, Nishida M, Ikenaga S, Hirata K, Zempo N, Esato K. (2002) Therapeutic angiogenesis induced by local autologous bone marrow cell implantation. Ann Thorac Surg 73:1210–1215.

Korbling M, Katz RL, Khanna A, Ruifrok AC, Rondon G, Albitar M, Champlin RE, Estrov Z. (2000) Hepatocytes and epithelial cells of donor origin in recipients of peripheral-blood stem cells. N Engl J Med 346:738–746.

Lagasse E, Connors H, Al-Dhalimy M, Reitsma M, Dohse M, Osborne L, Wang X, Finegold M, Weissman IL, Grompe M. (2000) Purified hematopoietic stem cells can differentiate into hepatocytes in vivo. Nat Med 6:1229–1234.

Lee KD, Kuo TK, Whang-Peng J, Chung YF, Lin CT, Chou SH, Chen JR, Chen YP, Lee OK. (2004) In vitro hepatic differentiation of human mesenchymal stem cells. Hepatology 40:1275–1284.

Muraca M, Gerunda G, Neri D, Vilei MT, Granato A, Feltracco P, Meroni M, Giron G, Burlina AB. (2002) Hepatocyte transplantation as a treatment for glycogen storage disease type Ia. Lancet 359:317–318.

Okabe M, Ikawa M, Kominami K, Nakanishi T, Nishimune Y. (1997) "Green mice" as a source of ubiquitous green cells. FEBS Lett 407:313–319.

Okamoto R, Yajima T, Yamazaki M, Kanai T, Mukai M, Okamoto S, Ikeda Y, Hibi T, Inazawa J, Watanabe M. (2002) Damaged epithelia regenerated by bone marrow-derived cells in the human gastrointestinal tract. Nat Med 8: 1011–1017.

Omori K, Terai S, Ishikawa T, Aoyama K, Sakaida I, Nishina H, Shinoda K, Uchimura S, Hamamoto Y, Okita K. (2004) Molecular signature associated with plasticity of bone marrow cell under persistent liver damage by self-organizing-map-based gene expression. FEBS Lett 578:10–20.

Petersen BE, Zajac VF, Michalopoulos GK. (1998) Hepatic oval cell activation in response to injury following chemically induced periportal or pericentral damage in rats. Hepatology 27:1030–1038.

Petersen BE, Bowen WC, Patrene KD, Mars WM, Sullivan AK, Murase N, Boggs SS, Greenberger JS, Goff JP. (1999) Bone marrow as a potential source of hepatic oval cells. Science 284:1168–1170.

Pittenger MF, Mackay AM, Beck SC, Jaiswal RK, Douglas R, Mosca JD, Moorman MA, Simonetti DW, Craig S, Marshak DR. (1999) Multilineage potential of adult human mesenchymal stem cells. Science 284:143–147.

Sakaida I, Terai S, Yamamoto N, Aoyama K, Ishikawa T, Nishina H, Okita K. (2004) Transplantation of bone marrow cells reduces CCl4-induced liver fibrosis in mice. Hepatology 40:1304–1311.

Schena M, Shalon D, Davis RW, Brown PO. (1995) Quantitative monitoring of gene expression patterns with a complementary DNA microarray. Science 270:467–470.

Shinoda K, Mori S, Ohtsuki T, Osawa Y. (1992) An aromatase-associated cytoplasmic inclusion, the "stigmoid body," in the rat brain: I. Distribution in the forebrain. J Comp Neurol 322:360–376.

Stamm C, Westphal B, Kleine HD, Petzsch M, Kittner C, Klinge H, Schumichen C, Nienaber CA, Freund M, Steinhoff G. (2003) Autologous bone-marrow stem-cell transplantation for myocardial regeneration. Lancet 361:45–46.

Tateishi-Yuyama E, Matsubara H, Murohara T, Ikeda U, Shintani S, Masaki H, Amano K, Kishimoto Y, Yoshimoto K, Akashi H, Shimada K, Iwasaka T, Imaizumi T. (2003) Therapeutic Angiogenesis using Cell Transplantation (TACT) Study Investigators. Therapeutic angiogenesis for patients with limb ischaemia by autologous transplantation of bone-marrow cells: a pilot study and a randomised controlled trial. Lancet 360:427–435.

Terada N, Hamazaki T, Oka M, Hoki M, Mastalerz DM, Nakano Y, Meyer EM, Morel L, Petersen BE, Scott EW (2002) Bone marrow cells adopt the phenotype of other cells by spontaneous cell fusion. Nature 416:542–545.

Terai S, Sakaida I, Yamamoto N, Omori K, Watanabe T, Ohata S, Katada T, Miyamoto K, Shinoda K, Nishina H, Okita K. (2003) An in vivo model for monitoring trans-differentiation of bone marrow cells into functional hepatocytes. J Biochem 134:551–558.

Theise ND, Nimmakayalu M, Gardner R, Illei PB, Morgan G, Teperman L, Henegariu O, Krause DS. (2000) Liver from bone marrow in humans. Hepatology 32:11–16.

Uchida N, Fujisaki T, Eaves AC, Eaves CJ. (2001) Transplantable hematopoietic stem cells in human fetal liver have a CD34(+) side population (SP)phenotype. J Clin Invest 108:1071–1077.

Vassilopoulos G, Wang PR, Russell DW. (2003) Transplanted bone marrow regenerates liver by cell fusion. Nature 422:901–904.

Vig P, Russo FP, Edwards RJ, Tadrous PJ, Wright NA, Thomas HC, Alison MR, Forbes SJ. (2006) The sources of parenchymal regeneration after chronic hepatocellular liver injury in mice. Hepatology 43:316–324.

Wang X, Willenbring H, Akkari Y, Torimaru Y, Foster M, Al-Dhalimy M, Lagasse E, Finegold M, Olson S, Grompe M. (2003) Cell fusion is the principal source of bone-marrow-derived hepatocytes. Nature 422:897–901.

Watanabe M. (2002) Damaged epithelia regenerated by bone marrow-derived cells in the human gastrointestinal tract. Nat Med 8:1011–1017.

Watanabe T, Nakagawa K, Ohata S, Kitagawa D, Nishitai G, Seo J, Tanemura S, Shimizu N, Kishimoto H, Wada T, Aoki J, Arai H, Iwatsubo T, Mochita M, Watanabe T, Satake M, Ito Y, Matsuyama T, Mak TW, Penninger JM, Nishina H, Katada T. (2002) SEK1/MKK4-Mediated SAPK/JNK Signaling Participates in Embryonic Hepatoblast Proliferation via a Pathway Different from NF-kappaB-Induced Anti-Apoptosis. Dev Biol 250:332–347.

Wexler SA, Donaldson C, Denning-Kendall P, Rice C, Bradley B, Hows JM. (2003) Adult bone marrow is a rich source of human mesenchymal "stem" cells but umbilical cord and mobilized adult blood are not. Br J Haematol 121:368–374.

Willenbring H, Bailey AS, Foster M, Akkari Y, Dorrell C, Olson S, Finegold M, Fleming WH, Grompe M. (2004) Myelomonocytic cells are sufficient for therapeutic cell fusion in liver. Nat Med 10:744–748.

Xiao L, Wang K, Teng Y, Zhang J. (2003) Component plane presentation integrated self-organizing map for microarray data analysis. FEBS Lett 538:117–124.

Yamamoto N, Terai S, Ohata S, Watanabe T, Omori K, Shinoda K, Miyamoto K, Katada T, Sakaida I, Nishina H, Okita K. (2004) A subpopulation of bone marrow cells depleted by a novel antibody, anti-Liv8, is useful for cell therapy to repair damaged liver. Biochem Biophys Res Commun 313:1110–1118.

Ying QL, Nichols J, Evans EP, Smith AG. (2002) Changing potency by spontaneous fusion. Nature 416:545–548.

Cryopreservation of hepatocytes -Is it effective to cryopreserved hepatocytes using a new cryopreservation procedure combining a bioartificial approach? -

Aoki T, Yasuda D, Enami Y Tomotake K, Izumida Y, Kusano T, Hayashi K, Odaira T, Yamada K, Murai N, Niiya T, Shimizu Y, Kusano M.

Department of Surgery, Division of Gastro-Intestinal Surgery, School of Medicine, Showa University, Tokyo, Japan, 142-8666.
1-5-8, Hatanodai, Shinagawa-ku, Tokyo, Japan.

Summary.

The number of patients with severe liver disease and needing whole organ transplantation or living related split liver transplantation has been increasing. However, the shortage of donor organs is particularly problematic and still awaits resolution.

Hepatocyte transplantation may serve as an alternative to organ transplantation for patients with life-threatening liver disease (te Velde AA et al, 1992, Ambrosino G et al. 2003, Strom SC et al. 1997, Fox IJ et al. 2004, Mito M et al 1992, Kusano M et al. 1981, Arkadopoulos et al. 1998). However, the application of allogeneic hepatocyte transplantation is also limited for the same reasons, lack of donors and poor proliferation of hepatocytes in vitro. It is desirable to establish a banking system of large quantities of hepatocytes allowing a large number of hepatocytes to be stored for a long time, thereby providing a convenient and easily accessible supply.

Cryopreservation is a standard technique for long-term storage of hepatocyes (Mirty RR, et al. 2002). However, standard cryopreservation procedures markedly injure hepatocytes. For several years, institutes have tried to devise new strategies for long term storage which would adequately protect hepatocytes (Lloyd TD et al, 2003). Although utilizing a programmable freezer with a special medium for cryopreservation was an effective and exciting method for cryopreservation of hepatocytes, new methods were still needed to avoid decreasing cell viability and maintaining various liver functions. We review here the traditional cryopreservation method and new cryopreservation procedures for hepatocyte which are based on combination with the bioartificial approach.

Key words. cryopreservation, hepatocytes, hepatocyte transplantation, alginate/poly-L/lysine

1. Standarization of hepatocyte cryopreservation

As for the principle of cell preservation, it is desirable to suppress cellular metabolic activity as much as possible during preservation, while maintaining the survival and function of the cell after thawing. As to long-term cryopreservation, liquid nitrogen is effective for preservation of isolated hepatocyte.

The problem of cryopreservation is ice crystal formation inside and outside of the cell produced at the time of freezing, and high salts which cause mechanical destruction of the cell membrane, or cell organella, and endocellular dehydration, as well as deformation and atrophy, etc. Although 1 and 2-propanediol (Rodrigues AP et al. 2004, Wusteman MC et al. 2002)), dextran (Halberstadt M et al. 2003, Halberstadt M et al. 2001), glycerol (Fuller BK et al. 2004), and DMSO (Sket P et al. 1995, Chense C et al, 1993, Loretz LJ et al. 1989, Gomez-Lechon MJ et al. 1984, Dou M et al. 1992, Son JH et al 2004) have been used as cryoprotectants, it turns out that glycerol is not suitable for hepatocytes (Fuller B et al. 1980, Kasai S et al. 1993). DMSO is most used widely at present. DMSO can delay ice crystal formation during the freezing process and cell injury is considered to be prevented as a result. Many investigators have shown the most suitable final concentration of DMSO to be 10 to 20% (Sket P et al. 1995, Chense C et al, 1993, Loretz LJ et al. 1989, Gomez-Lechon MJ et al. 1984, Dou M et al. 1992, Son JH et al 2004). Although Hengstler reported freezing speed and DMSO concentration in detail, a 10% DMSO concentration is the optimal, and further gradual addition of DMSO appeared to be required (Hengster JG et al. 2000). Guillouzo demonstrated that the best results were obtained with a 16% DMSO concentration for rat hepatocytes, 14% for other animal parenchymal cells and 10-12% for human hepatocytes (Guillouzo A et al. 1999).

Extracellular-macromolecules, particularly at serum concentrations between 10-20% v/v have also been included in addition to the DMEM, presumably to minimize osmotic shock during thawing. However, higher serum concentrations do not improve cell-viability or recovery. On the other hand, Muller demonstrated that primary porcine hepatocytes were frozen and maintained their specific liver functions without serum in liquid nitrogen by using a computer-assisted freezing device (Muller P et al. 2004).

Although there are protocols which employ a programming freezer in the freezing process slow cooling rates (between 1 °C/min to -10 °C/min) have generally been used to intermediate subzero temperatures (-60 °C to -80 °C) and before transfer to liquid nitrogen.

Quick thawing is another dangerous step, which again causes cell injury. To carry out quick thawing and to remove the cryoprotectant quickly, are both very important for assuring good subsequent viability. Quick thawing is performed in a 37 °C warm water bath in many protocol (Sket P et al. 1995, Chense C et al, 1993, Loretz LJ et al. 1989, Gomez-Lechon MJ et al. 1984, Dou M et al. 1992, Sun JH et al 2004).

As noted above, it is common to use DMSO as cryoprotectant and to freeze slowly using a programming freezer when hepatocytes are cryopreserved. At the time of thawing, quick thawing is carried out using a 37 °C warm water bath, and with these procedures, a high rate of survival can be achieved.

2 . Development of a new cryopreservation procedure combining a bioartificial approach

An detailed examination of the cell functional maintenance after freezing / thawing is made by combining the cryopreservation liquid or programming freezer has been reported until now. Recently, some investigators have succeeded in applying this new cryopreservation procedure which combines bioartificial material to avoid injury with ice crystal formation in frozen cells. The physiological and morphological function of a cell can be maintained by culturing cells in a three-dimensional structure (3D). Koebe developed a method to cryopreserve porcine hepatocytes immobilized in collagen gel on a tissue culture surface (Koebe et al. 1996). Cells were cultured for 3days prior to cryopreservation. Linear cooling was either at -1 °C /min or rapid at -10 °C /min to -80 °C. They also used slow cooling which was interrupted at -30 °C and the rate was then increased to -10 °C to -80 °C. The best recoveries were noted when these interrupted

24

cooling regimes were used, but even in these cases a post-thaw culture period of several days was needed to restore activity (19).

Dixit and Guymard reported an encapsulation technique using alginate beads gel to be useful and beneficial for cryopreservation of hepatocytes (Guyomard C et al. 1996, Dixit V et al. 1993). The semipermeable membrane of encapsulated cells allows the free exchange of oxygen, nutrients and metabolites but excludes the passage of immunocytes, antibodies and complement factors. Dixit showed that microencapsulation provides protection against the body's immune mechanisms, and may also provide for a favorable environment for the long-term well-being of hepatocytes. They demonstrated isolated hepatocytes to be encapsulated via a certain alginate/poly-L-lysine method, and they mixed the preparation with 10% DMSO, 20% FBS, and 70% RPMI, preserved it at -70 °C for 24 hours, and succeeded in cryopreservation within the liquid nitrogen. Furthermore, the encapsulated hepatocytes after freezing/thawing, are transplanted into Gunn rats which show hyperbilirubinemia. The bilirubin value improvement was maintained for 30 days after transplantation (Dixit V et al. 1993). Guyomard demonstrated the effectiveness of hepatocyte cryopreservation using encapsulation technique. They evaluated that survival and a variety of functions including various phase I and phase II enzyme activities in alginate-entrapped rat hepatocytes before and after cryopreservation and showed that all of the functions tested were well-preserved after freezing and thawing (Guyomard C et al. 1993).

The authors reported that encapsulation of human and rat hepatocytes was carried out in cryopreservation-medium consisting of 80% DMEM, 10% FBS and 10% DMSO. Encapsulated hepatocytes were distributed in freezing vials and immediately transferred to liquid nitrogen and stored. Placing the vials in a warm water bath at 37 °C thawed the encapsulated hepatocytes. This system is extremely simple and inexpensive, and moreover is a universal method. With our freeze-thaw protocol, cell viability, organic anion transporter expression and drug-metabolizing enzyme expression of entrapped hepatocytes were well preserved after a various time points of cryopreservation, and that the entrapped hepatocytes retained a normal appearance and well-preserved nuclei after 90 days of cryopreservation. Cryopreserved encapsulated human hepatocytes also retained viability and hepatic function similar to that of cryopreserved encaspsulated rat hepatocytes (Aoki T et al. 2005).

Encapsulated hepatocytes were generally limited by low mechanical strength, long-term degeneration of the capsule, and frequent induction of inflammatory responses. As mentioned above, one important advantage of encapsulation is the protection it provides for hepatocytes during cryopreservation processes. Canaple demonstrated that a new system, based on polyelectrolyte complexation between sodium alginate, cellulose sulphate and poly (methylene-co-guanidine) hydrochloride (PMCG), has important properties promoting cell encapsulation (Canaple et al. 2001). They demonstrated murine hepatocytes to be encapsulated in these capsules. The cryopreservation of encapsulated hepatocytes for periods of up to 4 months did not alter their functional activities and no major differences were observed between unfrozen and frozen encapsulated cells for the functions tested.

A very important subject in regards to establishing a better hepatocyte storage method is examining the synergistic effects with a cryopreservation procedure which uses bioartificial materials. Furthermore, the freezing / thawing speed protocol currently used must be examined in greater detailed. Kuleshova demonstrated that optimization of the procedure and solutions allow microencapsulated hepatocytes to be preserved with almost 100% retention of cell functions and no detectable damage to the fragile microcapsules (Kuleshova LL et al. 2004). They reported the optimal vitrification solution to consist of 40% ethylene glycol and 0.6M sucrose and that three cooling rates (400 degree C/min and above) and three warming rates (650 degree C/min and above), in combination with the proposed vitrification solution, were equally effective.

5 Conclusions

Hepatocyte transplantation is anticipated to be available for various liver diseases in the near future. Thus, the demand for hepatocyte will increase further. Assuming such a situation, raises concerns about the shortage of fresh hepatocytes, and heralds a rapid increase in the demand for frozen hepatocytes. Therefore, it is essential to develop methods of storing large number of hepatocytes without lost of their liver specific functions. For several years, investigators have attempted to devise new strategies for long term storage which would adequately protect hepatocytes as stated above. We strongly believe that our new technology for cryopreservation of hepatocytes combing bioartificial approach, which is based on traditional procedure for hepatocyte cryopreservation, will accelerate efforts to achieve hepatocyte transplantation as a clinical option in the near future.

This work was supported in part by a Showa University Grant-in Aid for Innovative Collaborative Research Projects and a special research Grant-in-Aid for Development of Characteristic Education from the Japanese Ministry of Education, Culture, Sports, Science and technology.

References

te Velde AA, Bosman DK, Oldenburg J, Sala M, Maas MA, Chamuleau RA. Three different hepatocyte transplantation techniques for enzyme deficiency disease and acute hepatic failure. Artif Organs 1992; 16: 522.

Ambrosino G, Varotto S, Basso SM, et al. Hepatocyte transplantation in the treatment of acute liver failure: microencapsulated hepatocytes versus hepatocytes attached to an autologous biomatrix. Cell Transplant 2003; 12: 43.

Strom SC, Fisher RA, Thompson MT, et al. Hepatocyte transplantation as a bride to orthotopic liver transplantation in terminal liver failure. Tranplantation 1997; 63: 559.

Fox IJ, Roy-Chowdhury J. Hepatocyte transplantation. J Hepatol 2004; 40: 878.

Mito M, Kusano M, Kawaura Y. Hepatocyte transplantation in Man. Transplant Proc. 1992; 24: 3052.

Kusano M, Ebata H, Mito M et al. Transplantation of cryopreserved isolated hepatocytes into rat spleen. Transplant Proc 1981; 13: 848-854.

Arkadopoulos N, Lilja H, Sub KS, Demetriou AA, Rozga J. Intrasplenic transplantation of allogeneic hepatocytes prolongs survival in anhepatic rats. Hepatology 1998; 28: 1365.

Mitry RR, Hughes RD, Dhawan A. progress in human hepatocytes: isolation, culture & cryopreservation. Semin Cell Dev Bio. 2002; 13: 463-467.

Lloyd TD, Orr S, Skett P, Berry DP, Dennison AR. Cryopreservation of hepatocytes: a review of current methods for banking. Cell tissue bank. 2003; 4: 3-15.

Rodrigues AP, Amorim CA, Costa SH, Matos MH, Santos RR, Lucci CM, Bao SN, Ohashi OM, Figueiredo JR. Cryopreservation of canine ovarian tissue using dimethylsulphoxide and propanediol. Anim Reprod Sci. 2004; 84: 211-227.

Wusteman MC, Pegg DE, Robinson MP, Wang LH, Fitch P. Vitrification media: Toxicity, permeability, and dielectric properties. Cryobiology. 2002; 44: 24-37.

Halberstadt M, Bohnke M, Athmann S, Hagenah M. Cryopreservation of human donor corneas with dextran. Invet Opthalmol Vis Sci. 2003; 44: 5110-5115.

Halberstadt M, Athmann S, Hagenah M. Corneal cryopreservation with dextran. Cryobiology. 2001; 43: 71-80.

Fuller BK. Cryoprotectants: the essential antifreezes to protect life in the frozen state. Cryo Letters. 2004; 25: 375-388.

Hengster JG, Ringel M, Biefang K, et al. Cultures with cryopreserved hepatocytes: applicability for studies of enzyme induction. Chem Biol Interact. 125: 51-73, 2000.

Madan A, Dehaan R, Carroll K, et al. Effect of cryopreservation on cytochrome P-450 enzyme induction in cultured rat hepatocytes. Drug Metab Disp. 1999; 27: 327-335.

Skett P, Tyson C, Guillouzo A, Maier P. Report on the international workshop on the use of human in vitro liver preparations to study drug metabolism in drug development. Biochem. Parmacol. 1995; 50: 280-285.

Chense C, Guyomard C, fautrel A, Poullain M.G., Fremond B, Jong H.De, Guillouzo A. Viability and function in primary culture of adult hepatocytes from various animal species and human being after cryoprerservation. Hepatology. 1993; 18: 406-414.

Loretz LJ, Li AP, Flye MW, Wilson AGE. Optimization of cryopreservation procedures for rat and human hepatocytes, Xenobiotica. 1989; 19: 489-498.

Gomez-Lechon MJ, Lopez P, Castell JV. Biochemical functionality and recovery of hepatocytes after deep freezing storage. In vitro. 1984; 20: 826-832.

Dou M, Sousa De, Lacarelle B, Placidi M, Lechene de la Porte P, Domingo M, Lafont H, Rahmani R. Thawed human hepatocytes in primary culture. Cryobiology. 1992; 29: 454-469.

Son JH, Kim KH, Nam YK, Park JK, Kim SK. Optimization of cryoprotectants for cryopreservation of rat hepatocyte. Biotechnol Lett. 2004; 26: 829-833.

Fuller B, Morris G, Attenburrow V, et al. Functional recovery of isolated rat hepatocytes from 196 °C. Cryo-Lett. 1980; 1: 139-146.

Kasai S, Mito M. Large scale cryopreservation of isolated dog hepatocytes. Cryobiology. 1993; 30: 1-11.

Guillouzo A, Rialland L, Fautrel A, Guyomard C. Survival and function of isolated hepatocytes after cryopreservation. 1999; 121: 7-16.

Guyomard C, Rialland L, Fremond B, Chense C, Guillouzo A. Infuluence of alginate gel entrapment and cryoprerservation on survival and xenobiotic metabolism capacity of rat hepatocytes. Toxicol Appl Pharmacol. 1996; 141: 349-356.

Koebe H, Dahnhardt C, Schilderg F et al. Cryopreservation of porcine hepatocytes. Cryobiology 1996; 33: 127-141.

Dixit V, Darvasi R, Arthur M, Lewin K, Gitnick G. Cryopreserved microencapsulated hepatocytes-transplantation studies in Gunn rats. Transplantation. 1993; 55: 616-622.

Canaple L, Nurdin N, Angelova N, Saugy D, Hunkeler D, Desvergne B. Maintenance of primary murine hepatocyte functions in multicomponent polymer capsules-in vitro cryopreservation studies. J Hepatology. 2001; 34: 11-18.

Kuleshova LL, Wang XW, Wu YN, Zhou Y, Yu H. Vitrification of encapsulated hepatocytes with reduced cooling and warming rates. Cryo-Lett. 2004; 25: 241-254.

Muller P, Aurich H, Wenkel R, Schaffner I, wolff I, Walldorf J, Fleig WE, Christ B. Serum-free cryopreservation of porcine hepatocytes. Cell Tissue Res. 2004; 317: 45-56.

Aoki T, Koizumi T, Kobayashi Y, et al. A novel method of cryopreservation of rat and human hepatocytes by using encapsulation technique and possible use for cell transplantation. Cell Transplant. 14; 2005, 609-620.

Induction of Hair Re-growth by Protein Kinase C η

Motoi Ohba

Institute of Molecular Oncology, Showa University, 1-5-8 Hatanodai, Shinagawa-ku, Tokyo 142-8555, Japan

Summary. Hair development is controlled by several families of signaling molecules, including Fgfs, Wnts and protein kinase Cs (PKC). Among PKC genes expressing in skin and hair follicle, the eta (η) isoform of PKC has been known to be a key regulator of the growth and differentiation of keratinocytes. We describe here that PKCη is involved in the hair cycle progression from telogen (quiescence phase) to anagen (growing phase). The hair re-growth was induced by a topical application of 12-*o*-tetradecanoylphorbol 13-acetate (TPA), a strong activator of PKC, on the dorsal skin of PKCη transgenic mice. The hair bulb grew down into the fatty tissue in PKCη transgenic mice after treatment of TPA, whereas it was located in the dermis in normal mice. Large amounts of the melanin accumulated in the hair follicles, indicating the initiation of anagen phase. Furthermore, introduction of PKCη by adenovirus vector into the skin of normal mice exhibited the remarkable newly hair growth. These findings might help to develop the novel chemical therapy for alopecia and establish the reconstitution of skin with hair follicles.

Keywords. PKC, hair growth

Introduction

Identification of molecules inducing hair growth contributes to the development of drugs for alopecia and the establishment of skin reconstitution with hair follicles. Previous studies propose the involvement of several factors in the hair induction, namely fibroblast growth factor, transforming growth factor, Wnt and protein kinase C (PKC) families (Oro 1998).

PKC comprises 11 members of isoforms with closely related structures. Each isoform possesses unique physiological features in the substrate specificity, mechanisms of up- or down-regulation and the subcellular localization (Nishizuka 1988). In epithelia, five isoforms of PKC are expressed: PKC α, δ, ε, η and ζ. Among them, PKCη is highly expressed in the differentiating and differentiated epithelial tissues (Osada 1993). Overexpression of PKCη induces the terminal differentiation of normal keratinocytes (Ohba 1998). PKCη transgenic mice display the hyperthickening of epidermis and the aberrant expression of epidermal specific proteins, indicating the acceleration of differentiation. However, little is known whether PKCη affects the hair growing and cell cycle progression of the hair follicle.

We present here that PKCη inducess the anagen entry of hair cycle and subsequent hair re-growth in mouse skin.

Materials and Methods

Topical application of phorbol ester

The hair of wild type C3H/HeN mice and PKC transgenic mice (7weeks age) in the second tologen phase of the hair cycle, was removed by hair clippers. One week later, TPA was topically applied onto the back skin.

Adenovirus gene transfer

Wild type C3H/HeN mice were anesthetized with pentobarbital (25mg / kg), and hair of backskin was shaved. Stratified Corneum was removed by the tape-stripping method. An eppendorf lid with a pinhole was then sealed to the skin by superglue. Adenoviruses (3.0 x 10^9 pfu) were injected into the lid using a 21-gauge needle and the lid was settled for 3hr.

Results

The hair cycle consists of three phases, i.e. anagen (growth phase), catagen (involution phase), telogen (rest/quiescence phase). To explore the function of PKCη in hair growth, we examined the effect of TPA on the hair re-growth of PKCη transgenic mice with the telogen phase of hair follicle. A low dose of TPA was topically applied onto the dorsal skin with hair follicles in the second telogen phase. After 12 days of treatment of 1n mole of TPA, new hair remarkably grew from skin surface of PKCη-transgenic mice, but not normal ones. The hair further grew by about 3 weeks after treatment of TPA, consequently the length was same as the unshaved hair (Fig. 1A). The hair exhibited the straight shape like a normal hair, but a little bit thinner.

Histopathological analysis shows that the hair follicle entered

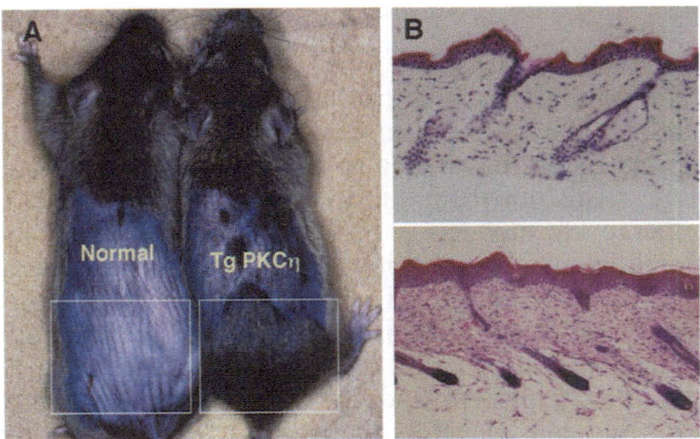

Fig. 1. Induction of anagen by a topical application of phorbolester in PKCη transgenic mice.   A.   TPA (1 n mole) in acetone was once applied on the back skin of normal mice or the PKCη transgenic mice (Tg PKCη), which were during the second telogen phase.   Open box shows the area of a TPA application.   B.   The H&E staining of the skin section of Tgη mice with TPA treatment.   The hair bulb expanded into the fatty tissue, indicating the induction of anagen. (Upper panel: Day1, Lower panel; Day 7)

the growing phase in the skin of the PKCη-transgenic mice. The hair bulb was located in dermis during the telogen of both normal and PKCη-transgenic mice.   However, the hair bulb grew down into the fatty tissue by TPA treatment only in Tg mice.   In addition, the melanin granules accumulated in the follicular papilla, being characteristic of the initiation of anagen (Fig. 1B).

Next, we introduced the PKCη-expressing adenovirus vector into the back skin of normal mice.   The hair expansion was apparently seen only in the area introduced PKCη adenovirus vector at 12 days after infection (Fig.2).   The hair growing continued by 16days (data not shown).   These results indicate that the activation and expression of PKC η initiate the anagen phase of hair cycle.

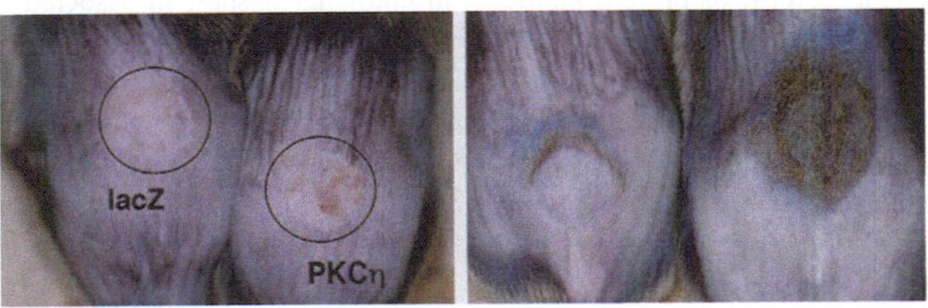

Fig. 2. Induction of hair regrowth by introducing PKCη with adenovirus vector..   PKCη adenovirus vector was infected into the back skin of C3H/HeN normal mice (7 weeks age).   Open circles show the area of infection.   The hair regrowth was observed in the area induced PKCη adenovirus vector.   The LacZ-expressing adenovirus vector was used as a negative control (Left panel: 2 days after infection, Right panel: 12 days).

Discussion

In present study, we found the acceleration of hair growth by PKCη. Phorbol ester including TPA has been known as an effective initiator of the hair cycle progression, but it is also a strong tumor promoter (Wilson et al. 1994). This drawback hinders the application of PKC activators on the therapy to alopecia. However, PKCη induces the keratinocytes differentiation and inhibits the skin tumor formation (Ohba et al. 1998, Chida et al. 2003). Therefore, there is a possibility that the PKCη-specific activator is utilized for the chemical therapy for alopecia as an effective and harmless drug. Further elucidation of the 3D structure of PKCη protein and the specific mechanism of activation needs to find and develop the specific activator(s) for PKCη.

Reference

Chida K, Hara T, Hirai T, Konishi C, Nakamura K, Nakao K, Aiba A, Katsuki M, Kuroki T. (2003) Disruption of protein kinase Cη results in impairment of wound healing and enhancement of tumor formation in mouse skin carcinogenesis. Cancer Res 63: 2404-2408

Nishizuka Y (1988) The molecular heterogeneity of protein kinase C and its implications for cellular regulation. Nature 334: 661-665

Ohba M, Ishino K, Kashiwagi M, Kawabe S, Chida K, Huh NH, Kuroki T. (1998) Induction of differentiation in normal human keratinocytes by adenovirus-mediated introduction of the η and δ isoforms of protein kinase C. Mol Cell Biol 18: 5199-5207

OroAE, Scott M.P (1998) Splitting hairs: dissecting roles of signaling systems in epidermal development. Cell 95: 575-578

Osada S, Hashimoto Y, Nomura S, Kohno Y, Chida K, Tajima O, Kubo K, Akimoto K, Koizumi H, Kitamura Y, Kuroki T(1993) Predominant expression of nPKCη, a Ca^{2+}-independent isoform of protein kinase C in epithelial tissues, in association with epithelial differentiation. Cell Growth Differ 4(3):167-75.

Wilson C, Cotsarelis G, Wei ZG, Fryer E, Margolis-Fryer J, Ostead M, Tokarek R, Sun TT, Lavker RM. (1994) Cells within the bulge region of mouse hair follicle transiently proliferate during early anagen: heterogeneity and functional differences of various hair cycles. Differentiation 55: 127-136

Novel Model for Evaluation of Human Skin Injury

Bunsho Kao , Yoshiyasu Amikura , Eri Honda , Yosuke Tomizuka , and Yoshiaki Hosaka

Department of Plastic and Reconstructive Surgery, Showa University School of Medicine, 1-5-8 Hatanodai, Shinagawa-ku, Tokyo 142-8666, Japan

Summary. In order to optimize wound healing of human skin, a method must be developed to reliably compare the potential for epidermal preservation and dermal fibroblast stimulation. We report a novel human skin tissue culture model developed for this purpose. An artificial skin model, consisting of human keratinocytes in the epidermis and human fibroblasts and rat-tail collagen in the dermis, was cultured using the floating collagen gel method. This model mimics in vivo human skin in terms of structure, cellular activity and function. Cultured fibroblasts form dense collagen fibrils, which repress fibroblast growth similar to that seen in vivo in the dermis. The keratinocyte layers on top of the dermal layer similarly mimic the epidermis of in vivo skin. Some laser irradiation and cryogen spray cooling exposure were applied to test the applicability of our model for characterization of epidermal and dermal wound healing.
We observed dynamic changes of the irradiated area on the artificial skin samples. Tissue regeneration can be clearly observed.
The model can be used to assess the potential for epidermal and dermal wound healing and offers several advantages over traditional animal and human skin models.

Key words. floating collagen gel, artificial human skin, laser skin resurfacing; photorejuvenation, cryogen injury

34

INTRODUCTION

Previous studies of wound healing involved either animal models or human subjects, but neither method is completely satisfactory. Rat or porcine skin is commonly used in animal studies, but the wound healing response in these models certainly differs from that of human skin after laser treatment. As a result, conclusions from such studies may not be relevant for human skin. In human studies, it is difficult to compare the effects of different devices or multiple irradiation parameters on a single subject. In addition, human studies are subject to concerns regarding post-irradiation medical care, cosmetic effects of biopsies, and regulatory obstacles. We propose an alternative model for objective in vitro evaluation of wound healing of human skin.

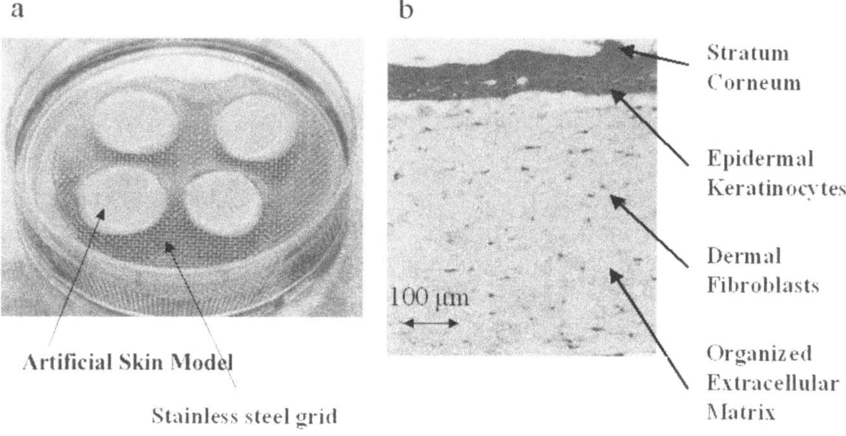

Fig. Artificial skin model (a) The model on a stainless steel grid in a culture dish; (b) Histopathology of the model. [Hematoxylin and eosin (H&E) stain; original magnification 100 X.].

MATERIALS AND METHODS

The discussed model is a form of artificial skin, composed of human keratinocytes in the epidermal layer, and human fibroblasts and rat-tail collagen in the dermal layer. Our model mimics in vivo human skin in terms of structure, cellular activity, and function. The keratinocyte layers on top of the dermal layer mimic the epidermis of in vivo human skin.

Cultured fibroblasts form dense collagen fibrils, which repress fibroblast growth, similar to that seen in vivo in the dermis.

STUDIES

Er:YAG laser irradiation study

In this study, we were able to preserve a thin layer of epidermis after sub-threshold Er:YAG laser irradiation. In addition, the average dermal fibroblast number was significantly increased at 1 week post-laser irradiation, relative to non-irradiated control samples harvested at the same time. [Kao B et al. (2003)] These results approach the goals of nonablative photorejuvenation: epidermal preservation and dermal fibroblast stimulation. The model offers a variety of benefits over previously utilized test media. This model mimics human skin better than animal models because it contains human keratinocytes and fibroblasts and also has human skin-like structure. Many identical specimens can be tested simultaneously without the difficulties and limitations inherent to animal and human studies. The model can be engineered as desired by varying the size, dermal thickness, and cell density. Further, there is the potential with this model, for manipulation of other factors relevant to the healing process including inflammatory cells, cytokines, and perhaps even blood flow.

Cryogen spray cooling exposure study

Cryogen spray cooling (CSC) is commonly used during dermatologic laser surgery. The epidermal and dermal effects of CSC have not been adequately evaluated. To study the potential for epidermal and dermal injury after CSC using an in vitro model of human skin, the specimens were exposed to continuous CSC spurt durations of 10, 20, 40, 80, 100, 200, or 500 milliseconds. [Kao B et al. (2004)] Biopsies were taken acutely, 3 and 7 days post-CSC exposure. Sections were stained with hematoxylin and eosin for evaluation of possible injury, Ki-67 to determine keratinocyte viability, and Melan-A, to identify and evaluate melanocytes. Minimal, transient epidermal changes were noted in specimens exposed to continuous CSC spurts of 80 milliseconds or less. Keratinocytes and melanocytes remained viable. Continuous CSC spurts of

100, 200, or 500 milliseconds (much longer than recommended for clinical use) resulted in significant epidermal injury acutely, with partial or full thickness epidermal necrosis at 7 days. Only the 500 milllisecond specimen demonstrated dermal change, decreased fibroblast proliferation at 3 days. ContinuousCSCspurts of 80 milliseconds or less induce minimal, if any, epidermal or dermal damage and are unlikely to produce cryo-injury when used during dermatologic laser surgery.

Perovskite laser irradiation with OCT monitoring study

An artificial skin model, which closely approximates human skin, was irradiated with a Perovskite laser ($\lambda = 1341$ nm) which is under investigation for potential use as a non-ablative laser skin rejuvenation device (NALSR).[Jung W et al. (2003)] Optical coherence tomography (OCT) was used to determine the extent of laser injury immediately post irradiation and, subsequently, to monitor tissue recovery over a 7-day period. OCT images clearly delineated areas of post-irradiation collagen injury and allowed non-invasive monitoring of the wound healing process. Histology was used for comparison and correlated well with OCT images. OCT offers advantages over standard histology as it is non-invasive and allows serial monitoring at the same site over time. Our results indicate that OCT has potential as a method for characterization of collagen injury post-laser irradiation and may be a useful tool for determination of optimal parameters for NALSR using different devices under investigation for this indication.

References

Jung W, Kao B, Kelly KM, Nelson JS, Chen Z (2003) Optical coherence tomography for in vitro monitoring of wound nealing after laser irradiation. IEEE Journal of selected topics in quantum electronics, 9(2) 1-4

Kao B, Kelly KM, Majaron B, J. Nelson JS (2003) Novel model for evaluation of epidermal preservation and dermal collagen remodeling following photorejuvenation of human skin. Lasers in Surgery and Medicine 32(2), 115–119

Kao B, Kelly KM, Aguilar G, Hosaka Y, Barr RJ, Nelson JS (2004) Evaluation of Cryogen Spray Cooling Exposure on In Vitro Model Human Skin. Lasers in Surgery and Medicine 34(2), 146–157

Heparin enhances BMP activity by maintaining high levels of nuclear phosphorylated Smad1/5/8

Baohong Zhao[1], Takenobu Katagiri[2], Hiromitsu Toyoda[3], Takatora Takada[4], Tatsuya Koike[3], Kunio Takaoka[3], Ryutaro Kamijo[1]

Departments of [1]Biochemistry and [4]Periodontology, School of Dentistry, Showa University, 1-5-8 Hatanodai, Shinagawa-ku, Tokyo 142-8555, Japan
[2] Division of Pathophysiology, Research Center for Genomic Medicine, Saitama Medical School, 1397-1 Yamane, Hidaka-shi, Saitama 350-1241, Japan
[3]Department of Orthopaedic Surgery, Osaka City University Medical School, 1-4-3 Asahimachi, Abenoku, Osaka 545-8585, Japan

Summary. Bone morphogenetic proteins (BMPs) inhibit myogenic differentiation and induce osteoblast differentiation in C2C12 myoblasts. Recently, we found that sulfated polysaccharides, including heparin, enhance the biological activities of BMPs. In this study, we examined the molecular mechanism by which heparin enhanced BMP activity. The mRNA levels of alkaline phosphatase and Osterix induced by BMP-2 were further increased in the presence of heparin. Phosphorylation of Smad1/5/8 was induced by BMP-2 within 1h, and heparin increased that at 24 hr. Most phosphorylated Smad proteins were localized in nuclei in the presence or absence of heparin. Although the concentration of BMP-2 in culture media sharply decreased to an undetectable level within 1 day in the absence of heparin, significantly higher levels of BMP-2 were detected in media in the presence of heparin. Taken together, these results suggest that heparin enhances BMP activity by maintaining high levels of nuclear phosphor-Smad 1/5/8 through maintaining active BMP-2 in culture media.

Key words. BMP, heparin, osteoblast differentiation, Smad 1/5/8

1 Introduction

BMPs, members of the TGF-beta superfamily, were originally identified because of their ability to induce ectopic bone formation when implanted into muscular tissues. Evidence has demonstrated that BMPs

38

are crucial molecules during normal bone development and osteoblast differentiation through the Smad signaling pathway (Katagiri et al., 2002). We previously reported that BMP-2 inhibits myogenic differentiation of C2C12 myoblasts and converts their differentiation pathway to that of osteoblast lineage cells (Katagiri et al., 1994). BMPs have osteogenic potential in vivo; therefore, they are of great interest as therapeutic agents for healing bone fractures, preventing osteoporosis and enhancing bone formation in bone defects. However, it has not been elucidated how to prolong the residence and efficacy of BMPs in local regions.

BMPs are sulfated polysaccharide-binding molecules because they were originally isolated by heparin affinity columns. Sulfated polysaccharides such as heparin and heparan sulfate are macromolecules associated with the cell surface. The extracelluar matrix and polysaccharides have been shown to interact directly with a number of growth factors, including BMPs, via highly negative-charged polysaccharide chains, and to affect their biological activities. Our recent results indicated that sulfated polysaccharides, including heparin, enhance the biological activities of BMPs (Takada et al., 2003), but the molecular mechanism of the stimulatory capacity of heparin is not clear.

In this study, we utilized C2C12 cells as the model for osteoblast differentiation and report that heparin enhances BMP activity by maintaining high levels of nuclear phosphor-Smads through maintaining active BMP-2 in culture media.

2 Materials and Methods
2.1 BMP and heparin
Purified recombinant human BMP-2 was obtained from Astellas Pharmaceuticals Co., Ltd. (Tokyo, Japan). Heparin prepared from porcine intestine was purchased from Sigma Chemical Co. (St. Louis, MO).
2.2 C2C12 Cell cultures for treatment with BMP-2
C2C12 cells were treated with heparin as described previously (Takada et al., 2003).
2.3 Reverse Transcription-Polymerase Chain Reaction
RT-PCR was performed as described previously (Yanai et al., 2001). The primers for each cDNA were as follows: ALP, GATCATTCCCACGTTTTCAC and TGCGGGCTTGTGGGACCTGC; Osterix, TTAAGCTTGCGTCCTCTCTGCTTGA and TTTCTAGATCAGATCTCTAGCAGGTT; GAPDH, TGAAGGTCGGTGTGAACGGATTGGC and CATGTAGGCCATGAGGTCCACCAC.
2.4 Immunohistochemical staining

Cells were immunohistochemically stained as described (Katagiri et al., 1994) using rabbit anti-Phospho-Smad1/5/8 antibody (Cell Signaling Technology, Inc. USA) and a Simple Stain AEC Solution Kit (HISTOFINE, Nichirei, Co.).

2.5 Western blot analysis

Western blot analysis was performed as described previously (Takada et al., 2003) using rabbit anti-phospho-Smad1/5/8 antibody and anti-Smad1 antibody (UPSTATE Biotechnology, NY).

2.6 ELISA for BMP-2

The BMP-2 concentrations in the culture media were quantitatively determined by ELISA using BMP-2 Immunoassay Kit (Quantikine, USA).

3 Results

First, we examined the effect of heparin on the gene expression related to osteoblast differentiation, such as alkaline phosphatase (ALP) and Osterix (Fig. 1). We observed that the mRNA level of ALP was further increased by heparin at 12, 24 and 72 hr. Heparin failed to enhance the mRNA level of Osterix, a key transcription factor for osteoblast differentiation, within 12 hr, but it increased those levels at 24 and 72 hr.

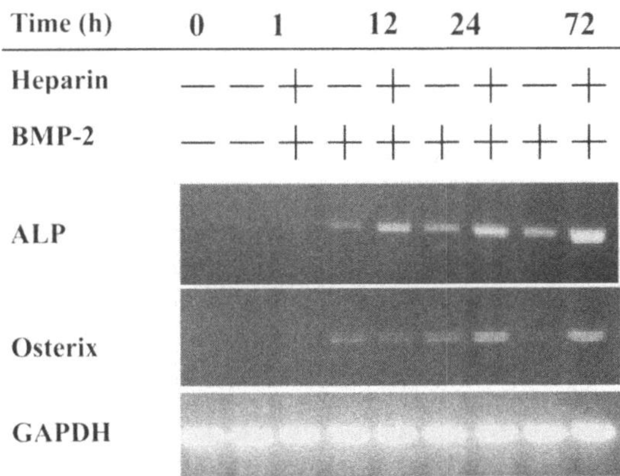

Fig. 1. Heparin enhances gene expression related to osteoblast differentiation induced by BMP-2 in C2C12 cells. C2C12 cells were incubated with 100ng/ml BMP-2 in DMEM containing 2.5% FBS with or without 5ug/ml heparin. Total RNAs were extracted at 0, 1, 12, 24 and 72hr. RT-PCR analysis was performed.

BMPs exert their biological activities by phosphorylating and activating intracellular Smad 1/5/8 transcription factors, which is a pivotal step in the BMP-2 signaling pathway. Upon BMP-2 stimulation, phosphorylated Smad proteins were accumulated in the nuclei within 1 hr in the presence and absence of heparin (Fig. 2). Most phosphorylated Smads disappeared at 24 hr in the absence of heparin. In contrast, heparin maintained phosphorylated Smads in the nuclei even at 24 hr. Western blot analysis also showed that heparin did not increase the phosphorylation of Smad1/5/8 stimulated by BMP-2 at 1 or 6 hr, whereas the levels of phosphorylated Smad 1/5/8 were enhanced by heparin at 24 hr (Fig. 3).

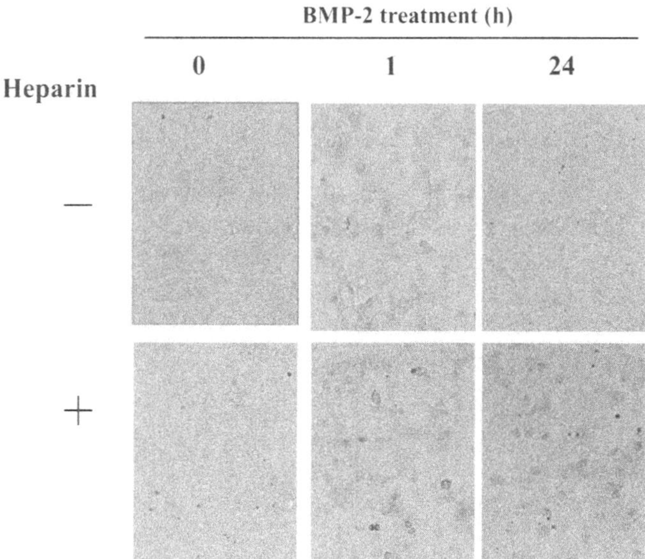

Fig. 2. Nuclear localization of phospho-Smad 1/5/8 induced by BMP-2. C2C12 cells were treated with 100 ng/ml BMP2 in DMEM containing 2.5% FBS in the presence or absence of 5ug/ml heparin over the time course (0, 1, and 24h), then immunochemistry staining was performed as described in Materials and Methods.

Fig. 3. Heparin enhances phosphorylation of Smad1/5/8 induced by BMP-2. C2C12 cells were treated with 100 ng/ml BMP2 in DMEM containing 2.5% FBS in the presence or absence of 5ug/ml heparin over the time course (0, 1,6 and 24 h), then Western blot analysis was performed as described in Materials and Methods.

Next, we quantified BMP-2 concentrations in culture media by ELISA (Fig. 4). The concentration of BMP-2 in culture media was sharply decreased to an undetectable level after 24 h in the absence of heparin. In contrast, significantly higher levels of BMP-2 were detected in the presence of heparin. These data indicated that heparin maintained BMP-2 concentration in the media.

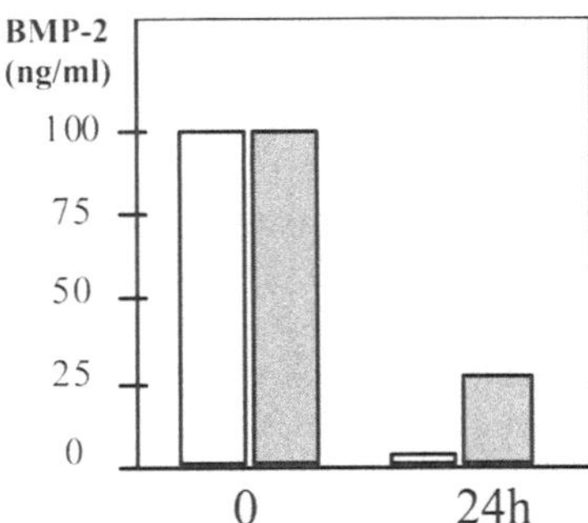

Fig. 4. Time-course changes in BMP-2 concentrations in culture media. C2C12 cells were treated with 100 ng/ml BMP2 in DMEM containing 2.5% FBS in the presence (solid bar) or absence (empty bar) of 5ug/ml heparin for 24h. BMP-2 concentrations in culture media were quantitatively determined by ELISA.

4 Discussion

It was revealed that sulfated polysaccharides, including heparin, enhance the biological activities of BMPs (Takada et al., 2004). In this study we showed that mRNA expression levels of ALP and Osterix, which are closely related to osteoblast differentiation, were also enhanced by heparin.

Smads are a conserved family of signal transducers of the TGF-β superfamily. Smad1, 5 and 8 are signaling molecules specific for the BMP pathway. Smad1, 5 and 8 are directly phosphorylated by BMP type I receptors and then translocated into the nucleus to regulate the transcription of various target genes. In the presence of dominant-negative Smads that block signaling, BMP-mediated effects are absent. In contrast, Smad overexpression enhances BMP signaling. Our work showed that heparin enhances the phosphorylation and nuclear accumulation of Smad1/5/8 induced by BMP-2, suggesting that the BMP signaling pathway was continuously enhanced in the presence of heparin.

Our previous study showed that heparin decreased the amount of ligand-receptor complex on C2C12 cell membranes (Takada et al., 2003). Furthermore, in this study, we found that the concentration of BMP-2 in the culture media was significantly higher in the presence than in the absence of heparin. Taken together, these results suggest that the BMP-2 ligand is maintained by heparin in the media and continuously serves as an active form to stimulate their receptors to continuously stimulate the intracellular signaling molecule Smad1/5/8. Moreover, our recent preliminary experiments showed that heparin significantly enhanced new bone formation induced by BMP-2 when heparin and BMP-2 were implanted together into muscle tissues in mice. Heparin enhances the biological activities of BMPs, offering a bright future to the clinical application of BMP-2.

5 References

Katagiri T, Takahashi N. (2002) Regulatory mechanisms of osteoblast and osteoclast differentiation. Oral Dis. 8(3):147-59

Katagiri T, Yamaguchi A, Komaki M, Abe E, Takahashi N, Ikeda T, Rosen V, Wozney JM, Fujisawa-Sehara A, Suda T. (1994) Bone morphogenetic protein-2 converts the differentiation pathway of C2C12 myoblasts into the osteoblast lineage. J Cell Biol. 127(6 Pt 1):1755-66

Nishimura R, Kato Y, Chen D, Harris SE, Mundy GR, Yoneda T. (1998) Smad5 and DPC4 are key molecules in mediating BMP-2-induced osteoblastic differentiation of the pluripotent mesenchymal precursor cell line C2C12. J Biol Chem. 273(4):1872-9

Takada, T., Katagiri, T., Ifuku, M., Morimura, N., Kobayashi, M., Hasegawa, K., Ogamo, A., Kamijo, R. (Boston, 2004) Enhancement of biological activity of BMP by heparin. In Biological Mechanisms of Tooth Movement and Craniofacial Adaptation, eds. Davidovitch and Mah, Harvard Society for the Advancement of Orthodontics , p197-203

Takada T, Katagiri T, Ifuku M, Morimura N, Kobayashi M, Hasegawa K, Ogamo A, Kamijo R. (2003) Sulfated polysaccharides enhance the biological activities of bone morphogenetic proteins. J Biol Chem. 278(44):43229-35

Yanai, T., Katagiri, T., Akiyama, S., Imada, M., Yamashita, T., Chiba, H., Takahashi, N., and Suda, T. (2001) Expression of mouse osteocalcin transcripts, OG1 and OG2, is differently regulated in bone tissues and osteoblast cultures. J. Bone Miner. Metab. **19**(6), 345-351

Part II
The Cardiovascular System

Vascular engraftment and repair by adult non-hematopoietic stem/progenitor cells

Jeffrey L. Spees

Department of Medicine, Cardiovascular Research Institute, Stem Cell Core, University of Vermont, 208 South Park Drive, Suite 2, Colchester, VT, 05446 USA

Summary. Recent advances in our understanding of adult non-hematopoietic stem/progenitor cell biology may lead to powerful new therapies for vascular repair and for the treatment of ischemic tissue injury. This chapter will provide an overview of several non-hematopoietic stem/progenitor cell types that engraft and contribute to the vasculature (mesenchymal stem cells, MSCs; endothelial and smooth muscle progenitor cells, EPCs and SPCs; adipose-derived stem cells, ADSCs; and cardiac stem cells, CSCs) and mechanisms of angiogenic and postnatal vasculogenic repair by adult stem/progenitor cells.

1 Mesenchymal stem cells from bone marrow

Non-hematopoietic bone marrow stem/progenitor cells that differentiate into multiple cell types are called mesenchymal stem cells, marrow stromal cells, or multipotent stromal cells (MSCs). They were first identified by Friedenstein and colleagues in the 1970s (Friedenstein et al. 1974a, 1974b, 1976). MSCs are commonly described as clonal, plastic adherent cells from bone marrow that are capable of differentiating into osteoblasts, adipocytes, and chondrocytes (Friedenstein et al. 1974a, Pereira et al. 1995, Prockop 1997, Pittenger et al. 1999, Sekiya et al. 2002). Recent work has demonstrated that MSCs are also capable of differentiation into endothelial cells (Oswald et al. 2004), smooth muscle cells (Kobayashi et al. 2004), and a variety of other cell types both *ex vivo* and *in vivo* (reviewed in Prockop 1997, Prockop et al. 2003, Gregory et al. 2005).

MSCs are localized in the bone marrow as vascular pericytes and as endosteal stromal cells that support hematopoiesis (Shi and Gronthos

2003, Muguruma et al. 2006). They can serve as feeder layers to support the *ex vivo* culture of hematopoietic stem/progenitor cells by providing extracellular matrix components, cytokines, and growth factors (Friedenstein et al. 1974a, Dexter et al. 1984). In addition to replacing dying or injured cells, the secretion of numerous angiogenic, mitogenic, and anti-apoptotic factors by MSCs under both normoxic and hypoxic/ischemic conditions is likely to play a key role in their ability to prevent or repair ischemic tissue injury (Kinnaird et al. 2004a, Nagaya et al. 2005). MSCs can augment collateral perfusion (Kinnaird et al. 2004b) and have been demonstrated to increase vascular density, cardiac function and to differentiate into vascular endothelial and smooth muscle cells in a model of chronic cardiac ischemia (Silva et al. 2005).

2 Adipose-derived stem cells

Multipotent MSC-like progenitor cells were first isolated from adipose tissue in 2001 (Zuk et al. 2001). Adipose-derived stem cells (ADSCs) are similar to bone marrow-derived MSCs and can differentiate into bone, fat, cartilage, and muscle (Zuk et al. 2002). Freshly isolated progenitor cells from the stromal-vascular fraction of human adipose tissue or lipoaspirates are reported to express the stem/progenitor cell surface marker CD34 (Miranville et al. 2004, Planat-Benard et al. 2004), whereas cultured ADSCs have variable expression of the sialomucin, depending on the growth medium (Zuk et al. 2002, Miranville et al. 2004).

The administration of ADSCs was reported to improve the survival and repair of ischemic hindlimbs in mice by ADSC differentiation into endothlelial cells (Miranville et al. 2004) and by the secretion of angiogenic and anti-apoptotic factors such as vascular endothelial growth factor (VEGF) and hepatocyte growth factor (HGF) (Nakagami et al. 2005, Rehman et al. 2006). The presence of MSCs in the stromal-vascular fraction of adipose tissue suggests that MSC-like cells may exist as pericytes or pericyte-like cells throughout the vasculature in all adult tissues. Thus, the artery wall has been found to be both a destination and a source for multipotent cells that give rise to cartilage, bone, fat, muscle and vascular tissue (reviewed in Abedin et al. 2004).

3 Endothelial and smooth muscle progenitor cells

Asahara et al. reported the isolation of endothelial progenitor cells (EPCs) from human peripheral blood in 1997. This discovery and others that followed support the theory of postnatal vasculogensis, i.e. the contribution of circulating (likely bone marrow-derived) cells to growing blood vessels.

Historically, EPCs and their origin have been difficult to define. There remains also some confusion in the literature regarding EPCs since there are cells with varying degrees of proliferative potential that can contribute to vascular endothelium: CECs, "circulating endothelial cells" that are mature non-proliferative endothelial cells that are shed from the vessel wall, EPCs, "endothelial progenitor cells" that are primitive $CD133^+/VEGFR-2^+$ cells that are either positive or negative for CD34; EOCs, "endothelial outgrowth cells" that express several endothelial cell antigens and that can divide extensively in culture, and $CD14^+/CD34^{low}$ cells that were reported to be the predominant circulating endothelial stem cells (Romagnani et al. 2005). Circulating EPCs with a phenotype of CD34-negative/$CD133^+/VEGFR-2^+$ are believed to be the most potent EPCs in terms of homing to vascular injury and engaging in vascular repair (Friedrich et al. 2006). Therefore, several possibly related cells from the bone marrow, the circulation, and the vessel wall itself can contribute to vascular endothelium (reviewed in Urbich et al. 2004, Ingram et al. 2005). Similar to *ex vivo* culture of bone marrow MSCs, the culture of and culture conditions for EPCs or related cells with endothelial potential may profoundly influence their ability to engraft and to repair blood vessels when administered *in vivo*.

The bone marrow appears to be the major source of circulating EPCs. Endothelial engraftment of bone marrow-derived endothelial cell precursors has been observed following bone marrow transplantation in both mouse and man (Bailey et al. 2004, Jiang et al. 2004). Of special note, single cell transplantation studies using single purified KLS hematopoietic stem cells ($c-kit^+/Sca-1^+/lin^-$ cells) indicates that at least some if not all primitive EPCs arise from an adult bone marrow-derived hemangioblast-like cell that is capable both of reconstituting the blood cell lineages and engaging in postnatal vasculogenesis (Bailey et al. 2004).

Smooth muscle progenitor cells (SPCs) can also be isolated from adult peripheral blood and cultured (Simper et al. 2002). Bone marrow-transplanted mouse hematopoietic stem cells (HSCs, KLS cells) were reported to give rise to smooth muscle cells in neointima and atherosclerotic plaques (Sata et al. 2002). Similarly, smooth muscle cells in human coronary atherosclerosis were reported to arise from progenitor cells administered at the time of marrow transplantation (Caplice et al. 2003). $CD14^+/CD105^+$ enriched cells that express alpha smooth muscle actin (α-SMA) were recently isolated from circulating human peripheral blood and were demonstrated to differentiate into contractile smooth muscle cells with characteristic SM markers *ex vivo*. Furthermore, the percentage of cells with this SPC phenotype were shown to significantly increase in numbers in the circulation of patients with coronary artery disease compared with peripheral blood counts from control subjects (Sugiyama et al. 2005).

4 Cardiac stem cells

Adult cardiac stem cells (CSCs) were first reported in 2002 by a pioneering research group led by Piero Anversa (Quaini et al. 2002). Because of the reduced capacity for the heart to repair itself relative to other organ systems (e.g. liver) and the long held view that postnatal cardiomyocytes are postmitotic cells, the existence of endogenous stem/progenitor cells for the adult heart has led to a "paradigm shift" in cardiac biology. CSCs are clonal, self-renewing, and multipotent. They produce multiple cardiac cell types such as cardiac myocytes, endothelial cells and smooth muscle cells. Thus far, CSCs or CSC-like cells have been isolated from the hearts of mice, rats, dogs, pigs, and humans (reviewed in Anversa et al. 2006). In the context of ischemic cardiac injury, CSCs contribute to myocyte replacement and to vasculogenesis *in vivo* (Beltrami et al. 2003).

It is not clear whether CSCs and other mesodermal stem/progenitor cells are related to bone marrow-derived MSCs. One hypothesis is that related progenitor cells in adult tissues are specified to preferentially differentiate into the cell types of the tissue in which they reside. The bone marrow may be a reservoir for non-hematopoietic progenitor cells that can replenish distal tissues during chronic tissue injury or following injury to the stem cell compartment of a given tissue (Prockop et al. 2003). Recently, cardiac side-population (SP) cells that efflux Hoechst dye have been shown to differentiate into functional cardiac myocytes (Pfister et al. 2005). Following myocardial infarction, bone marrow-derived SP cells were observed to migrate to the injured heart and to undergo phenotypic conversion to cells with a cardiac SP immunophenotype (Mouquet et al. 2005); these data support the bone marrow "reservoir" hypothesis.

5 Mobilization and engraftment of adult stem/progenitor cells

Most adult non-hematopoietic progenitor cells share at least some aspects of ligand/receptor interactions for mobilization and engraftment during tissue injury. In particular, stromal-derived factor 1 (SDF-1) and VEGF, both released by ischemic tissues, are known to recruit multiple stem/progenitor cell types from the circulation and the bone marrow.

Currently, there is relatively incomplete knowledge regarding the mechanisms of bone marrow-derived or adipose-derived MSC mobilization. Results from several laboratories indicate that MSCs possess the receptors CXCR4 and CX3R1 and migrate in response to SDF-1 and fractalkine both *ex vivo* and *in vivo* (Wynn et al. 2004, Ji et al. 2004, Son et al. 2006, Lee et al. 2006). MSCs also express the c-met receptor and migrate on a gradient of HGF (Son et al. 2006). Adipose-derived MSCs were reported to migrate in culture in response to platelet-derived growth factor (PDGF-BB) via c-Jun N-terminal kinase (JNK) signaling (Kang et al. 2005).

EPCs are mobilized by a variety of secreted factors such as granulocyte monocyte-colony stimulating factor (GM-CSF), granulocyte-colony stimulating factor (G-CSF), SDF-1, erythropoietin (EPO), VEGF, and Angiopoietin-1 (reviewed in Aicher et al. 2005). In addition, EPCs can be mobilized pharmacologically by HMG-CoA reductase inhibitors (statins) in rodents (Dimmeler et al. 2001) and in patients (Vasa et al. 2001). EPCs can also be mobilized into the circulation during physical exercise (Laufs et al. 2004). Aside from mobilizing factors, adhesive proteins such as β2-integrins (Chavakis et al. 2005) and matrix degrading proteins such as cathepsin L (Urbich et al. 2005) are important for adhesive interactions with the vessel wall and EPC invasion.

Similar to bone marrow MSCs, cardiac stem cells express c-met receptors and migrate on a gradient of HGF. Importantly, HGF can be used to attract CSCs to sites of cardiac injury such as zones of infarction (Urbanek et al. 2005).

6 Vascular progenitors in vascular disease and repair

Under different disease conditions adult non-hematopoietic stem/progenitor cells repair the vasculature, while in other cases these cells may act pathologically. EPCs are mobilized following acute myocardial infarction (Shintani et al. 2001) and are believed to be beneficial for the repair of ischemic cardiac injury. EPCs and SPCs are known to engraft atherosclerotic plaques (Sata et al. 2002, George et al. 2005), but it is not entirely clear under which circumstances these cells contribute to plaque stabilization or to plaque vulnerability. Similar with the contribution of circulating fibrocytes to fibrosis, the contribution of vascular progenitor cells to atheroscleroisis may likely represent an attempt to repair disease rather than to promote it.

Adult bone marrow-derived non-hematopoietic progenitor cells have been shown to participate in vascular remodeling in the lungs of mice with hypoxia-induced pulmonary hypertension (PH) (Hayashida et al. 2005).

50

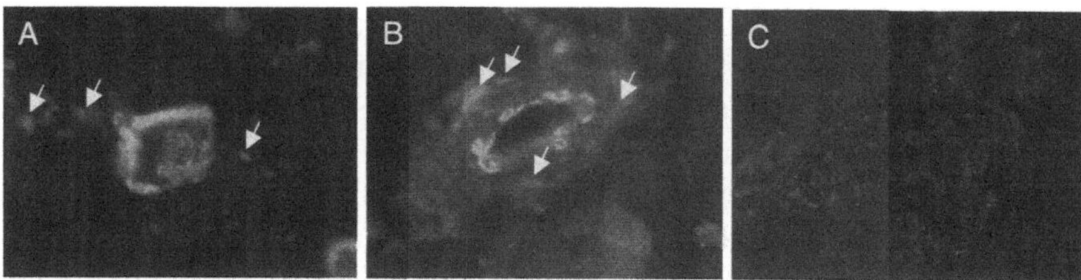

Fig. 1. Bone marrow progenitor cells participate in repair/remodeling during monocrotaline-induced pulmonary hypertension. A) Lung section from a control rat that received BMT but no MCT (6 weeks after BMT). Green (ALEXA 488): α-SMA staining of a blood vessel. Red (ALEXA 594): antibody staining of GFP-positive bone marrowderived cells. B) GFP-positive bone marrow cells (red) surround a blood vessel of a MCT-treated chimeric rat (6 weeks after BMT, 3 weeks after MCT). C) Y chromosome in situ hybridization (pink dots) to confirm the engraftment of male bone marrow-derived cells in the female host. Blue nuclei are stained with DAPI. Please refer also to the color plate in the front of this book.

EPO signaling has recently been demonstrated to be a critical component in the homing of EPCs to the lungs of mice with PH (Satoh et al. 2006). EPCs can ameliorate or rescue monocrotaline (MCT)-induced pulmonary hypertension when modified to express adrenomedullin or eNOS, possibly by protecting endothelial cells against apoptosis (Nagaya et al. 2003, Zhao et al. 2005).

In a bone marrow transplant/monocrotaline model of progressive pulmonary hypertension, we have observed that significant numbers of bone marrow-derived cells and non-hematopoietic progenitor cells engraft the lungs of rats and engage in repair/remodeling (Fig. 1). For the experiments, adult Female Sprague Dawley rats received bone marrow transplants (BMT) from transgenic GFP male Sprague Dawley rats. Three weeks after BMT, chimeric rats were injected intravenously with the alkaloid plant toxin monocrotaline (MCT). The metabolite of MCT causes progressive pulmonary hypertension. The animals were examined 3 weeks after MCT injection to allow the chronic injury (PH) to draw cells from the circulation and the bone marrow. We observed engraftment of both EPCs and SPCs in the lungs and hearts of chimeric rats (data not shown).

Reduced circulating EPC numbers or defects in mobilization are believed to negatively impact the prognosis of patients with cardiovascular disease. Impaired signaling of CXCR4 through Janus kinase in the EPCs of patients with coronary artery disease is likely to lead to reduced homing of EPCs and reduced neovascularization capacity (Walter et al. 2005). Patients with low circulating levels of EPCs may have greater risk for cardiovascular events (Schmidt-Lucke et al. 2005) and vasculopathy (Simper et al. 2003).

A decrease in circulating EPCs has also been shown to be associated with acute stroke patients and those with stable stroke compared with control subjects. Low levels of EPCs correlated inversely with the Framington risk factor score, indicating that EPC levels may be a predictive marker for vascular dysfunction (Ghani et al. 2004).

Supported by NIH grant HL077570-01 (to J.S.).

References

Abedin M, Tintut Y, Demer LL (2004) Mesenchymal stem cells and the artery wall. Circ Res 95:671–676

Aicher A, Zeiher AM, Dimmeler S (2005) Mobilizing endothelial progenitor cells. Hypertension 45:321–325

Anversa P, Kajstura J, Leri A, Bolli R (2006) Life and death of cardiac stem cells: a paradigm shift in cardiac biology. Circulation 113:1451–1463

Asahara T, Murohara T, Sullivan A, Silver M, van der Zee R, Li T, Witzenbichler B, Schatteman G, Isner JM (1997) Isolation of putative progenitor endothelial cells for angiogenesis. Science 275:964–967

Bailey AS, Jiang S, Afentoulis M, Baumann CI, Schroeder DA, Olson SB, Wong MH, Fleming WH (2004) Transplanted adult hematopoietic stems cells differentiate into functional endothelial cells. Blood 103:13–19

Beltrami AP, Barlucchi L, Torella D, Baker M, Limana F, Chimenti S, Kasahara H, Rota M, Musso E, Urbanek K, Leri A, Kajstura J, Nadal-Ginard B, Anversa P (2003) Adult cardiac stem cells are multipotent and support myocardial regeneration. Cell 114:763–776

Caplice NM, Bunch TJ, Stalboerge PG, Wang S, Simper D, Miller DV, Russell SJ, Litzow MR, Edwards WD (2003) Smooth muscle cells in human coronary atherosclerosis can originate from cells administered at marrow transplantation. Proc Natl Acad Sci USA 100:4754–4759

Chavakis E, Aicher A, Heeschen C, Sasaki K, Kaiser R, El Makhfi N, Urbich C, Peters T, Scharffetter-Kochanek K, Zeiher AM, Chavakis T, Dimmeler S (2005) Role of beta2-integrins for homing and neovascularization capacity of endothelial progenitor cells. J Exp Med 201:63–72

Dexter TM, Spooncer E, Schofield R, Lord BI, Simmons P (1984) Haemopoietic stem cells and the problem of self-renewal. Blood Cells 10:315–339

Dimmeler S, Aicher A, Vasa M, Mildner-Rihm C, Adler K, Tiemann M, Rutten H, Fichtlscherer S, Martin H, Zeiher AM (2001) HMG-CoA reductase inhibitors (statins) increase endothelial progenitor cells via the PI 3-kinase/Akt pathway. J Clin Invest 108:391–397

Friedenstein AJ, Chailakhyan RK, Latsinik, NV, Panasyuk, AF, Keiliss-Borok IV (1974a) Stromal cells responsible for transferring the microenvironment of the hemopoietic tissues. Cloning in vitro and retransplantation in vivo. Transplantation 17:331–340

Friedenstein AJ, Deriglasova UF, Kulagina NN, Panasuk AF, Rudakowa SF, Luria EA, Ruadkow IA (1974b) Precursors for fibroblasts in different

52

populations of hematopoietic cells as detected by the in vitro colony assay method. Exp Hematol 2:83–92

Friedenstein AJ, Gorskaja U, Kalugina NN (1976) Fibroblast precursors in normal and irradiated mouse hematopoietic organs. Exp Hematol. 4:267–274

Friedrich EB, Walenta K, Scharlau J, Nickenig G, Werner N (2006) CD34–/CD133+/VEGFR-2+ endothelial progenitor cell subpopulation with potent vasoregenerative capacities. Circ Res 98:e20–e25

George J, Afek A, Abashidze A, Shmilovich H, Deutsch V, Kopolovich J, Miller H, Keren G (2005) Transfer of endothelial progenitor and bone marrow cells influences atherosclerotic plaque size and composition in apolipoprotein E knockout mice. Arterioscler Thromb Vasc Biol 25:2636–2641

Ghani U, Shuaib A, Salam A, Nasir A, Shuaib U, Jeerakathil T, Sher F, O'Rourke F, Nasser AM (2004) Endothelial progenitor cells during cerebrovascular disease. Stroke 36:151–153

Gregory CA, Prockop DJ, Spees JL (2005) Non-hematopoietic bone marrow stem cells: Molecular control of expansion and differentiation. Exp Cell Res 306:330–335

Hayashida K, Fujita J, Miyake Y, Kawada H, Ando K, Ogawa S, Fukuda K (2005) Bone marrowderived cells contribute to pulmonary vascular remodeling in hypoxia-induced pulmonary hypertension. Chest 127:1793–1798

Ingram DA, Caplice NM, Yodar MC (2005) Unresolved questions, changing definitions, and novel paradigms for defining endothelial progenitor cells. Blood 106:1525–1531

Ji JF, He BP, Dheen ST, Tay SS (2004) Interactions of chemokines and chemokine receptors mediate the migration of mesenchymal stem cells to the impaired site in the brain after hypoglossal nerve injury. Stem Cells 22:415–427

Jiang S, Walker L, Afentoulis M, Anderson DA, Jauron-Mills L, Corless CL, Fleming WH (2004) Transplanted human bone marrow contributes to vascular endothelium. Proc Natl Acad Sci U S A 2004 Nov 30;101(48):16891–16896

Kang YJ, Jeon ES, Song HY, Woo JS, Jung JS, Kim YK, Kim JH (2005) Role of c-Jun N-terminal kinase in the PDGF-induced proliferation and migration of human adipose tissue-derived mesenchymal stem cells. J Cell Biochem 95:1135–1145

Kinnaird T, Stabile E, Burnett MS, Lee CW, Barr S, Fuchs S, Epstein SE (2004a) Marrowderived stromal cells express genes encoding a broad spectrum of arteriogenic cytokines and promote in vitro and in vivo arteriogenesis through paracrine mechanisms. Circ Res 94:678–685

Kinnaird T, Stabile E, Burnett MS, Shou M, Lee CW, Barr S, Fuchs S, Epstein SE (2004b) Local delivery of marrow-derived stromal cells augments collateral perfusion through paracrine mechanisms. Circulation 109:1543–1549

Kobayashi N, Yasu T, Ueba H, Sata M, Hashimoto S, Kuroki M, Saito M, Kawakami M (2004) Mechanical stress promotes the expression of smooth muscle-like properties in marrow stromal cells. Exp Hematol 32:1238–1245

Laufs U, Werner N, Link A, Endres M, Wassmann S, Jurgens K, Miche E, Bohm M, Nickenig G (2004) Physical training increases endothelial progenitor cells, inhibits neointima formation, and enhances angiogenesis. Circulation. 109:220–226

Lee RH, Hsu SC, Munoz J, Jung JS, Lee NR, Pochampally R, Prockop DJ (2006) A subset of human rapidly self-renewing marrow stromal cells preferentially engraft in mice. Blood 107:2153–2161

Miranville A, Heeschen C, Sengenes C, Curat CA, Busse R, Bouloumie A (2004) Improvement of postnatal neovascularization by human adipose tissue-derived stem cells. Circulation 110:349–355

Mouquet F, Pfister O, Jain M, Oikonomopoulos A, Ngoy S, Summer R, Fine A, Liao R (2005) Restoration of cardiac progenitor cells after myocardial infarction by self-proliferation and selective homing of bone marrow-derived stem cells. Circ Res 97:1090–1092

Muguruma Y, Yahata T, Miyatake H, Sato T, Uno T, Itoh J, Kato S, Ito M, Hotta T, Ando K (2006) Reconstitution of the functional human hematopoietic microenvironment derived from human mesenchymal stem cells in the murine bone marrow compartment. Blood. Mar 1;107(5):1878–1887. Epub 2005 Nov 10.

Nagaya N, Kangawa K, Kanda M, Uematsu M, Horio T, Fukuyama N, Hino J, Harada-Shiba M, Okumura H, Tabata Y, Mochizuki N, Chiba Y, Nishioka K, Miyatake K, Asahara T, Hara H, Mori H (2003) Hybrid cell-gene therapy for pulmonary hypertension based on phagocytosing action of endothelial progenitor cells. Circulation 108:889–895

Nagaya N, Kangawa K, Itoh T, Iwase T, Murakami S, Miyahara Y, Fujii T, Uematsu M, Ohgushi H, Yamagishi M, Tokudome T, Mori H, Miyatake K, Kitamura S (2005) Transplantation of mesenchymal stem cells improves cardiac function in a rat model of dilated cardiomyopathy. Circulation 112:1128–1135

Nakagami H, Maeda K, Morishita R, Iguchi S, Nishikawa T, Takami Y, Kikuchi Y, Saito Y, Tamai K, Ogihara T, Kaneda Y (2005) Novel autologous cell therapy in ischemic limb disease through growth factor secretion by cultured adipose tissue-derived stromal cells. Arterioscler Thromb Vasc Biol 25:2542–2547

Oswald J, Boxberger S, Jorgensen B, Feldmann S, Ehninger G, Bornhauser M, Werner C (2004) Mesenchymal stem cells can be differentiated into endothelial cells in vitro. Stem Cells 22:377–384

Pereira RF, Halford KW, O'Hara MD, Leeper DB, Sokolov BP, Pollard MD, Bagasra O, Prockop DJ (1995) Cultures of adherent cells from marrow can serve as long-lasting precursor cells for bone, cartilage and lung in irradiated mice. Proc Natl Acad Sci USA 92:4857–4861

Pfister O, Mouquet F, Jain M, Summer R, Helmes M, Fine A, Colucci WS, Liao R (2005) CD31– but Not CD31+ cardiac side population cells exhibit functional cardiomyogenic differentiation. Circ Res 97:52–61

Pittenger MF, Mackay AM, Beck SC, Jaiswal RK, Douglas R, Mosca JD, Moorman MA, Simonetti DW, Craig S, Marshak DR (1999) Multilineage potential of adult human mesenchymal stem cells. Science 284:143–147

Planat-Benard V, Silvestre JS, Cousin B, Andre M, Nibbelink M, Tamarat R, Clergue M, Manneville C, Saillan-Barreau C, Duriez M, Tedgui A, Levy

B, Penicaud L, Casteilla L (2004) Plasticity of human adipose lineage cells toward endothelial cells: physiological and therapeutic perspectives. Circulation 109:656–663

Prockop DJ (1997) Marrow stromal cells as stem cells for non-hematopoietic tissues. Science 276:71–74

Prockop DJ, Gregory CA, Spees JL (2003) One strategy for cell and gene therapy: harnessing the power of adult stem cells to repair tissues.Proc Natl Acad Sci U S A 100 Suppl 1:11917–11923

Quaini F, Urbanek K, Beltrami AP, Finato N, Beltrami CA, Nadal-Ginard B, Kajstura J, Leri A, Anversa P (2002) Chimerism of the transplanted heart. N Engl J Med 346:5–15

Rehman J, Traktuev D, Li J, Merfeld-Clauss S, Temm-Grove CJ, Bovenkerk JE, Pell CL, Johnstone BH, Considine RV, March KL (2004) Secretion of angiogenic and antiapoptotic factors by human adipose stromal cells. Circulation. 109:1292–1298

Romagnani P, Annunziato F, Liotta F, Lazzeri E, Mazzinghi B, Frosali F, Cosmi L, Maggi L, Lasagni L, Scheffold A, Kruger M, Dimmeler S, Marra F, Gensini G, Maggi E, Romagnani S (2005) CD14+CD34low cells with stem cell phenotypic and functional features are the major source of circulating endothelial progenitors. Circ Res 97:314–322

Sata M, Saiura A, Kunisato A, Tojo A, Okada S, Tokuhisa T, Hirai H, Makuuchi M, Hirata Y, Nagai R (2002) Hematopoietic stem cells differentiate into vascular cells that participate in the pathogenesis of atherosclerosis. Nat Med 8:403–409

Satoh K, Kagaya Y, Nakano M, Ito Y, Ohta J, Tada H, Karibe A, Minegishi N, Suzuki N, Yamamoto M, Ono M, Watanabe J, Shirato K, Ishii N, Sugamura K, Shimokawa H (2006) Important role of endogenous erythropoietin system in recruitment of endothelial progenitor cells in hypoxia-induced pulmonary hypertension in mice. Circulation 113:1442–1450

Schmidt-Lucke C, Rössig L, Fichtlscherer S, Vasa M, Britten M, Kämper U, Dimmeler S, Zeiher AM (2005) Reduced number of circulating endothelial progenitor cells predicts future cardiovascular events. Proof of concept for the clinical importance of endogenous vascular repair. Circulation 111:2981–2987

Sekiya I, Vuoristo JT, Larson BL, and Prockop DJ (2002) In vitro cartilage formation by human adult stem cells from bone marrow stroma defines the sequence of cellular and molecular events during chondrogenesis. Proc Natl Acad Sci USA 99:4397–4402

Shi S, Gronthos S (2003) Perivascular niche of postnatal mesenchymal stem cells in human bone marrow and dental pulp. J Bone Miner Res 18: 696–704

Shintani S, Murohara T, Ikeda H, Ueno T, Honma T, Katoh A, Sasaki K, Shimada T, Oike Y, Imaizumi T (2001) Mobilization of endothelial progenitor cells in patients with acute myocardial infarction. Circulation 103:2776–2779

Silva GV, Litovsky S, Assad JA, Sousa AL, Martin BJ, Vela D, Coulter SC, Lin J, Ober J, Vaughn WK, Branco RV, Oliveira EM, He R, Geng YJ, Willerson JT, Perin EC (2005) Mesenchymal stem cells differentiate into an endothelial phenotype, enhance vascular density, and improve heart function in a canine chronic ischemia model. Circulation 111:150–156

Simper D, Stalboerger PG, Panetta CJ, Wang S, Caplice NM (2002) Smooth muscle progenitor cells in human blood. Circulation 106:1199–1204

Simper D, Wang S, Deb A, Holmes D, McGregor C, Frantz R, Kushwaha SS, Caplice NM (2003) Endothelial progenitor cells are decreased in blood of cardiac allograft patients with vasculopathy and endothelial cells of non-cardiac origin are enriched in transplant atherosclerosis. Circulation 107:143–149

Son BR, Marquez-Curtis LA, Kucia M, Wysoczynski M, Turner AR, Ratajczak J, Ratajczak MZ, Janowska-Wieczorek A (2006) Migration of bone marrow and cord blood mesenchymal stem cells in vitro is regulated by SDF-1-CXCR4 and HGF-c-met axes and involves matrix metalloproteinases. Stem Cells [Epub ahead of print]

Sugiyama S, Kugiyama K, Nakamura S, Kataoka K, Aikawa M, Shimizu K, Koide S, Mitchell RN, Ogawa H, Libby P (2005) Characterization of smooth muscle-like cells in circulating human peripheral blood. Atherosclerosis

Urbanek K, Rota M, Cascapera S, Bearzi C, Nascimbene A, De Angelis A, Hosoda T, Chimenti S, Baker M, Limana F, Nurzynska D, Torella D, Rotatori F, Rastaldo R, Musso E, Quaini F, Leri A, Kajstura J, Anversa P (2005) Cardiac stem cells possess growth factor-receptor systems that after activation regenerate the infarcted myocardium, improving ventricular function and long-term survival. Circ Res 97:663–673

Urbich C, Dimmeler S (2004) Endothelial progenitor cells. Characterization and role in vascular biology. Circ Res 95:343–353

Urbich C, Heeschen C, Aicher A, Sasaki K, Bruhl T, Farhadi MR, Vajkoczy P, Hofmann WK, Peters C, Pennacchio LA, Abolmaali ND, Chavakis E, Reinheckel T, Zeiher AM, Dimmeler S (2005) Cathepsin L is required for endothelial progenitor cell-induced neovascularization. Nat Med 11: 206–213

Vasa M, Fichtlscherer S, Adler K, Aicher A, Martin H, Zeiher AM, Dimmeler S (2001) Increase in circulating endothelial progenitor cells by statin therapy in patients with stable coronary artery disease. Circulation 103: 2885–2890

Walter DH, Haendeler J, Reinhold J, Rochwalsky U, Seeger F, Honold J, Hoffmann J, Urbich C, Lehmann R, Arenzana-Seisdesdos F, Aicher A, Heeschen C, Fichtlscherer S, Zeiher AM, Dimmeler S (2005) Impaired CXCR4 signaling contributes to the reduced neovascularization capacity of endothelial progenitor cells from patients with coronary artery disease. Circ Res 97:1142–1151

Wynn RF, Hart CA, Corradi-Perini C, O'Neill L, Evans CA, Wraith JE, Fairbairn LJ, Bellantuono I (2004) A small proportion of mesenchymal stem cells strongly expresses functionally active CXCR4 receptor capable of promoting migration to bone marrow. Blood 104:2643–2645

Zhao YD, Courtman DW, Deng Y, Kugathasan L, Zhang Q, Stewart DJ (2005) Rescue of Monocrotaline-Induced Pulmonary Arterial Hypertension Using Bone Marrow-Derived Endothelial-Like Progenitor Cells. Efficacy of Combined Cell and eNOS Gene Therapy in Established Disease. Circ Res 96:442–450

Zuk PA, Zhu M, Mizuno H, Huang J, Futrell JW, Katz AJ, Benhaim P, Lorenz HP, Hedrick MH (2001) Multilineage cells from human adipose tissue: implications for cell-based therapies. Tissue Eng 7:211–228

Zuk PA, Zhu M, Ashjian P, De Ugarte DA, Huang JI, Mizuno H, Alfonso ZC, Fraser JK, Benhaim P, Hedrick MH (2002) Human adipose tissue is a source of multipotent stem cells. Mol Biol Cell 13:4279–4295

Importance of Neutrophil and Erythroblast for the efficacy of Bone-marrow Cell Implantation in Peripheral Artery Disease

Hiroshi Suzuki[1], Yoshitaka Iso[1], Taro Kusuyama[1], Yasutoshi Omori[1], Teruko Soda[1], Takatoshi Sato[1], Fumiyoshi Tsunoda[1], Makoto Shoji[1], Shinji Koba[1], Eiichi Geshi[1], Takashi Katagiri[1], Shigeru Tomoyasu[2]

[1]Third Department of Internal Medicine and [2]Department of Hematology, Showa University School of Medicine, 1-5-8 Hatanodai, Shinagawa-ku, Tokyo 142-8666, Japan

Summary. [Background] Efficacy of autologous bone marrow-mononuclear cell (BM-MNC) implantation as therapeutic angiogenesis has been reported in patients with severe peripheral artery disease. In addition to containing CD34 positive-cells, sorted BM-MNCs contain an abundance of CD34-negative cells. No studies have yet elucidated which types of CD34-negative cells influence the clinical appearance in BM-MNC implantation. We investigated the correlations of morphologically classified cell types of sorted BM-MNCs with changes in the ankle brachial index (ABI) and transcutaneous oxygen pressure (TcO_2). [Material and Methods] Seven patients with severe peripheral arterial disease who were not candidates for angioplasty or surgical operation underwent BM-MNC implantation. The sorted BM-MNCs using a cell separator were classified on the basis of May-Giemsa staining, and CD34-positive cells were counted. ABI and TcO_2 were performed before and after BM-MNC implantation. [Results] Mean ABI ($p<0.05$) and mean TcO_2 ($p<0.005$) from baseline to 4 weeks after the implantation were significantly increased. The numbers of total injected cells and CD34-positive cells were not correlated with ΔTcO_2 from before to 4 weeks. Among the cell types analyzed, ΔTcO_2 showed significant negative correlations with the percentage of mature neutrophils ($p<0.01$) and significant positive correlations with the percentage of erythroblasts ($p<0.05$). [Conclusions] Neutrophils could be an inverse regulator and erythroblasts could be a positive regulator in clinical BM-MNC implantation.

Key Words. Bone-marrow, Cell implantation, Neutrophil, Erythroblast, Peripheral artery disease

Autologous bone marrow-mononuclear cells (BM-MNC) implantation into ischemic limbs has recently been developed as a therapeutic angiogenesis for patients with severe peripheral artery disease without indications of percutaneous transluminal angioplasty or bypass surgery (Tateishi-Yuyama et al. 2002). In theory, the commitment of CD34-positive endothelial progenitor cells (EPC) to vessel formation, so-called vasculogenesis, is thought to be the main mechanism behind the angiogenic effect (Asahara et al. 1997). However, CD34-positive cells make up only a very small population among the BM-MNCs. As it turns out, sorted BM-MNC fraction contains not only CD34-positive cells, but also an abundance of CD34-negative cells of various types and differential grades. For this reason, closer investigation into the role of CD34-negative cells is very important to improve BM-MNC implantation. No previous reports have shown which types of blood cells influence the clinical appearance in patients treated by the BM-MNC implantation for ischemic limbs. Therefore, we investigated the correlations of morphologically classified cell types among sorted BM-MNCs with changes in ankle brachial index (ABI) and transcutaneous oxygen pressure (TcO$_2$) as clinical parameters of effectiveness in BM-MNC implantation.

Methods

Patients

Study subjects included 7 patients with peripheral arterial disease (7 men; mean age 61.6±7.9 years) who had symptoms of chronic limb ischemia such as severe intermittent claudication, rest pain, or non-healing ulcers, but who were not candidates for angioplasty or surgical operation. We excluded patients with poorly controlled diabetes mellitus (hemoglobin A1c>6.5% and proliferative retinopathy) or with evidence of a malignant disorder during the past 5 years. The study protocol was approved by the Ethics Committee of the Showa University. Written informed consent was obtained from all patients.

Methods

BM-MNCs

The procedure of BM-MNC implantation was previously described (Tateishi-Yuyama et al. 2002). After aspirating the bone marrow (about 600 ml) from the ileum under general anesthesia, the BM-MNCs were sorted on a CS3000-Plus blood-cell separator (Baxter International Inc., Deerfield, IL, USA), and concentrated to 60 ml. The separated cells were implanted into the ischemic legs by intramuscular injection.

A BM-MNC-floating solution after separation was used as smear sample,. The sorted BM-MNCs were classified on the basis of May-Giemsa staining. CD34-positive cells were counted using a fluorescence-activated cell sorter (FACS). The drugs used were not changed throughout the study.

ABI and TcO2

Oscillometric blood pressure in the ankle and brachium were measured using form PWV/ABI (Colin Co., Ltd, Komaki, Japan) before and 4 weeks after the implantation. The ABI was defined as the ratio of ankle systolic pressure to brachial systolic pressure (normal value>1.0).

TcO_2 was measured in a supine position at room temperature using an oxymonitor (tina TCM 4, Radiometer, Copenhagen, Denmark) (normal value>60 mmHg) before and 4 weeks after the implantation.

Changes in ABI and TcO2 between before and 4 weeks after the implantation were defined as ΔABI and ΔTcO2.

Statistical analyses

All values are expressed as mean$\pm$SD. Changes in variables from baseline to 4 weeks were analyzed with paired t test. The correlation coefficients between two variable parameters were determined by Peasons' simple linear regression analysis. Statistical significance was accepted at p<0.05.

Results

The characteristics of each patient are shown in Table.

Table: Patients' characteristics

Case	Age	Gender	Diagnosis	Fontaine	Previous therapy	HT	DM	HL	Smoking	HD
1	55	M	ASO	III	bypass	+	-	-	+	-
2	63	M	ASO	IV	bypass	+	-	-	+	-
3	70	M	ASO	III	bypass	-	+	-	-	-
4	47	M	Burger	IV	-	-	-	-	+	-
5	67	M	ASO	III	-	+	+	-	+	+
6	65	M	ASO	III	-	+	+	-	+	+
7	64	M	ASO	III	-	-	+	-	+	+

M, male; ASO, arteriosclerosis obliterans; HT, hypertension; DM, diabetes mellitus; HL, hyperlipidemia; HD, hemodialysis

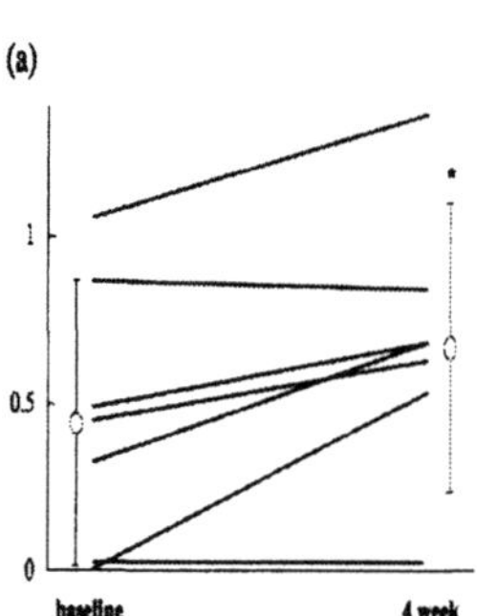

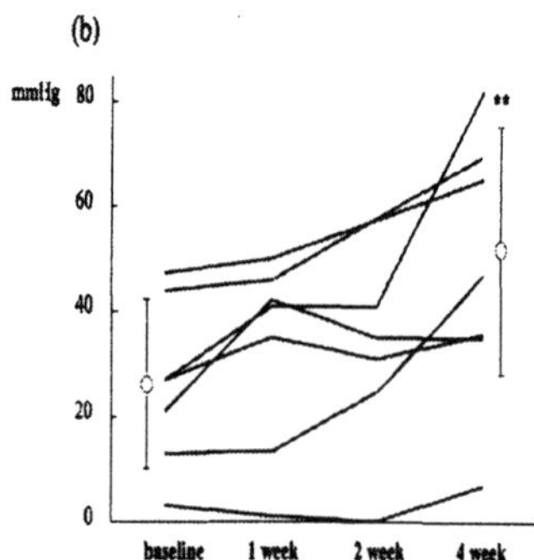

Figure 1: Changes in clinical parameters between baseline and 4 weeks after bone-marrow mononuclear cell implantation
(a) ankle brachial index (ABI) (b) transcutaneous oxygen pressure (TcO2)
* p<0.05, ** p<0.005

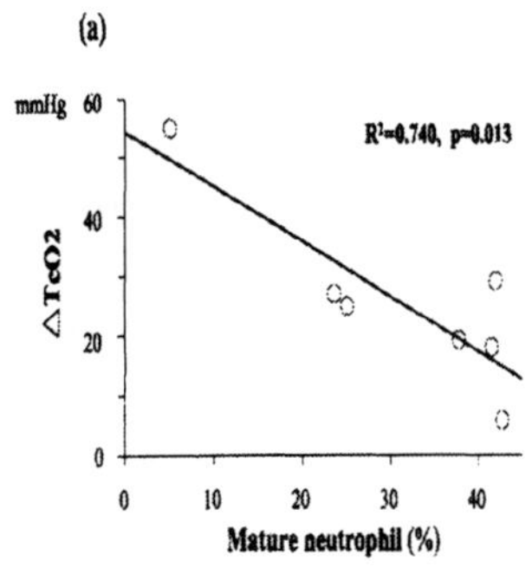
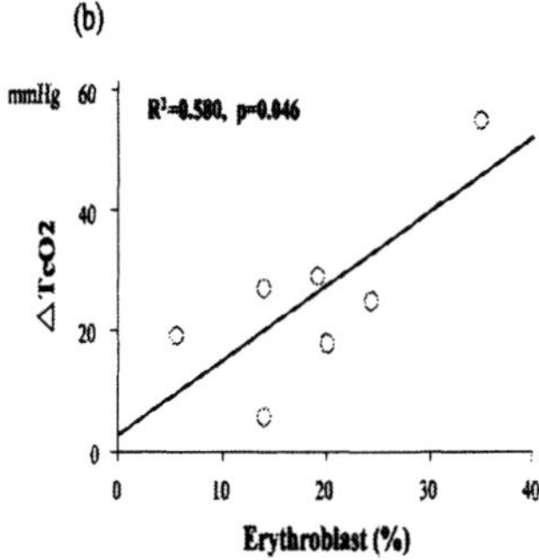

Figure 2:
Correlation between changes in transcutaneous oxygen pressure (TcO2) and percentage of injected cell types
(a) mature neutrophils (b) erythroblasts

Injected BM-MNCs

The mean number (SD) of injected cells was $3.3 \pm 0.8 \times 10^9$. The injected BM-MNCs included lymphocytoid cells (mean (SD) $26.5 \pm 11.4\%$), monocytoid cells ($7.8 \pm 4.6\%$), myeloblasts ($1.0 \pm 0.7\%$), myelocytes ($10.7 \pm 6.3\%$), mature neutrophils ($31.0 \pm 14.0\%$), and erythroblasts ($18.7 \pm 9.3\%$). The mean number of CD34-positive cells in FACS analysis was $3.1 \pm 1.4 \times 10^7$ ($0.9 \pm 0.3\%$ of the injected cells).

ABI, TcO2

ABI at 4 weeks after the implantation was higher than that at baseline in 5 out of 7 patients. The mean ABI at 4 weeks was significantly higher than that at baseline (0.38 ± 0.4 vs. 0.69 ± 0.4, p<0.05)(Figure 1a).
TcO_2 at 4 weeks after the implantation was higher than that at baseline in all patients. The mean TcO_2 at 4 weeks was significantly increased than that at baseline (25.0 ± 15.6vs 50.6 ± 24.3, p<0.005)(Figure 1b).

ABI and injected cell types

The numbers of total injected cells and CD34-positive cells were not correlated with ΔABI (the change of values from baseline to follow-up). The percentage of CD34-positive cells among the total injected cells also showed no correlation with ΔABI. In fact none of the morphologically classified cell types correlated with ΔABI on a percentage basis.

TcO2 and injected cell types

The numbers of total injected cells and CD34-positive cells were not correlated with ΔTcO$_2$ (the change of values from baseline to follow-up). The percentage of CD34-positive cells among the total injected cells also showed no correlation with ΔTcO$_2$. Among the morphologically classified cell types, mature neutrophils showed strongly significant negative correlations with ΔTcO$_2$ on a percentage basis (p=0.013, r=0.740, Figure 2a). On one hand, the erythroblasts showed significant positive correlations with ΔTcO$_2$ on a percentage basis (p=0.046, r=0.580, Figure 2b).

Discussion

The present study demonstrated significant increases in both TCO$_2$ and ABI from baseline to 4 weeks after BM-MNC implantation, showing the efficacy of this therapy.

While the numbers of injected nucleated cells and CD34-positive cells were not correlated with ΔTCO$_2$ or ΔABI, the percentages of mature neutrophils and erythroblasts showed a strongly significant negative correlation with ΔTCO$_2$ and a significant positive correlation with ΔTCO$_2$, respectively.

CD34-positive cells and efficacy of BM-MNC implantation

The correlation between the number of CD34-positive cells and ΔABI established in earlier research suggests that the number of implanted CD34-positive cells is one of the primary factors influencing the efficacy of BM-MNC implantation (Saigawa et al. 2004). However, our data showed that the number and percentage of CD34-positive cells implanted had no correlations with ΔTcO_2 or ΔABI. Our findings indicate that the efficacy of BM-MNC implantation depends not only on the number of CD34-positive cells, but also various other factors produced by CD34-negative cells. It has been reported that co-culture of human CD34-positive and CD34-negative MNCs yielded a greater number of EPCs than culture of CD34-positive MNCs alone, suggesting that intercellular communication between CD34-positive MNCs and CD34-negative cells is important for the differentiation of EPCs (Asahara et al.1997, Murohara et al. 2000).

Neutrophil and efficacy of BM-MNC implantation

Activated neutrophils have the potential to mediate endothelial injury by releasing lysosomal proteinases or generating oxygen metabolites. The present study showed that the percentage of neutrophils within the injected BM-MNCs was negatively correlated with ΔTcO_2, suggesting that the neutrophils are an important culprit in attenuating the efficacy of the therapeutic angiogenesis. Iba et al. also demonstrated that neutrophils had an inhibitory effect on angiogenesis and that neutrophil elastase contributed to the anti-angiogenic effect (Iba et al. 2002). We surmise that the therapeutic effects of BM-MNC implantation can be best improved by suppressing the anti-angiogenic factors in neutrophils such as neutrophil elastase.

Erythroblast and efficacy of BM-MNC implantation

Bone marrow erythroblasts have been reported to serve angiogenic factors, such as vascular endothelial growth factor A (VEGF-A) and placental growth factor (PlGF), possibly by acting as paracrine manner on monocyte/macrophages and /or endothelial cells (Tordjman et al. 2001). Erythroid cells have been reported to promote angiogenesis through the activation of VEGF and PlGF, and erythropoietin enhances this effect (Ozawa et al. 2004). Erythroblasts made up 18.7% of the injected cells in the present study and this percentage proved to be positively correlated with ΔTcO_2. We surmise that the therapeutic effects of BM-MNC implantation can be best improved by enhancing the pro-angiogenic factor in erythroblasts such as VEGF and PlGF.

Acknowledgments

We wish to thank to Prof. Tadanori Kawada from the First Department of Surgery at the Showa University School of Medicine for their kind guidance.

Conclusions

This study indicated that neutrophils could be an inverse regulator and erythroblasts could be a regulator in clinical BM-MNC implantation.

References

Asahara T, Murohara T, Sullivan A, Silver M, van der Zee R, Li T, Witzenbichler B, Schatteman G, Isner J (1997) Isolation of putative progenitor endothelial cells for angiogenesis. Science 275:964-967

Iba O, Matsubara H, Nozawa Y, Fujiyama S, Amano K, Mori Y, Kojima H, Iwasaka T (2002) Angiogenesis by implantation of peripheral blood mononuclear cells and platelets into ischemic limbs. Circulation 106:2019-2025

Murohara T, Ikeda H, Duan J, Shintani S, Sasaki K, Eguchi H, Onitsuka I, Matsui K, Imaizumi T (2000) Transplanted cord blood –derived endothelial precursor cells augment postnatal neovascularization. J Clin Invest 105:1527-1536

Ozawa T, Kato K, Saigawa T, Makiyama Y, Minagawa S, Watanabe R, Tsuchida K, Nakamura Y, Hanawa H, Kodama M, Aizawa Y (2004) Erythropoiesis induced angiogenesis in vitro. Circ J 68 (Suppl I):294

Saigawa T, Kato K, Ozawa T, Toba K, Makiyama Y, Minagawa S, Hashimoto S, Furukawa T, Nakamura Y, Hanawa H, Kodama M, Yoshimura N, Fujiwara H, Namura O, Sogawa M, Hayashi J, Aizawa Y (2004) Clinical application of bone marrow implantation in patients with arteiosclerosis obliterans, and the association between efficacy and the number of implanted bone marrow cells. Circ J 68:1189-1193

Tateishi-Yuyama E, Matsubara H, Murohara T, Ikeda U, Shintani S, Masaki H, Amano K, Kishimoto Y, Yoshimoto K, Akashi H, Shimada K, Iwasaka T, Imaizumi T (2002) Therapeutic angiogenesis for patients with limb ischaemia by autologous transplantation of bone-marrow cells: a pilot study and a randomized controlled trial. Lancet 360:427-435

Tordjman R, Delaire S, Plouet J, Ting S, Gaulard P, Fichelson S, Romeo PH, Remarchandel V (2001) Lemarchandel V. Erythroblasts are a source of angiogenic factors. Blood 97:1968-1974

Bone marrow derived cells contribute to arterial remodeling

Makoto Shoji, Hiroshi Suzuki, Taro Kusuyama, Yasutoshi Omori, Teruko Soda, Fumiyoshi Tsunoda, Takatoshi Sato, Shinji Koba, Eiichi Geshi, Takashi Katagiri

Third Department of Internal Medicine, Showa University School of Medicine, 1-5-8 Hatanodai, Shinagawa-ku, Tokyo 142-8555, Japan

Summary. Exuberant smooth muscle cells hyperplasia is the major cause of postangioplasty restenosis. We suggested that circulating smooth muscle progenitor cells might contribute to lesion formation after vascular injury. We extensively investigated the cellular constituents during neointimal formation after mechanical injury. A large wire was inserted into the mouse femoral artery. At 2 hours, the injured artery remained dilated with a thin media containing very few cells. One week after the injury, CD45 positive hematopoietic cells accumulated at the luminal side. Those CD 45 positive cells gradually disappeared, whereas neointimal was formed with alpha smooth muscle actin positive cells. Bone marrow cells and peripheral mononuclear cells differentiated into alpha smooth muscle cells in the presence of PDGF and basic FGF. These results suggest that early accumulation of hematopoietic cells may play a role in the pathogenesis of smooth muscle cells hyperplasia under certain circumstances.

Key words. Bone marrow derived cells, arterial remodeling

1 Introduction

As a future approach to improve the prognosis in such patients, investigations have recently Percutaneous coronary intervention (PCI) has been widely adopted as a treatment of atherosclerosis. However, in a significant number of patients, the procedure fails due to progressive vessel narrowing, or post-PCI restenosis (Nobuyoshi 1988). The pathogenesis of restenosis is multi-factorial, but abnormal hyperplasia of vascular smooth muscle cells (SMCs) is a common feature of post-PCI restenosis (Nobuyoshi 1991, Kearney M 1997). Recently, we suggested that bone marrow cells could give rise to vascular progenitor cells that potentially contribute to pathological remodeling in models of hyperlipidemia-induced atherosclerosis, post-PCI restenosis, and transplant-associated arteriosclerosis (Saiura 2001, Sata 2002, 2003). However, little is known about the mechanism by which bone marrow-derived cells participate in neointimal formation. Here, we extensively characterized cellular constituents during neointimal hyperplasia after mechanical vascular injury. Moreover, we examined whether bone marrow-derived cells differentiate into SMC like-cells *in vitro* and *in vivo*. Results document deposition of fibrin and platelets at the injured artery, followed by homing of hematopoietic cells and subsequent SMC hyperplasia, providing further insights into the mechanisms by which bone marrow-derived progenitor cells contribute to vascular repair and remodeling.

2 Method

2.1 Animal experimental protocol

Adult male 16- to 24-week-old inbred wild-type mice (C3H/He) weighing between 25 and 35 g. Transluminal mechanical injury of the femoral artery was induced by insertion of a large wire (0.38 mm in diameter) as previously described (Sata 2000). The mice were euthanized by intraperitoneal administration of an overdose of Nembutal at the time points indicated. At death, the mice were perfused with 0.9% NaCl solution followed by perfusion fixation with 4% paraformaldehyde in PBS (pH 7.4). Cross-sections (5 mm) were stained with hematoxylin and eosin.

2.2 Immunohistochemistry

Paraffin-embedded sections (5 μm) were deparaffinized, blocked with 0.5% goat serum, and incubated with an anti-mouse CD45 antibody (clone 30-F11, BD Pharmingen). Antibody distribution was visualized by the avidin-biotin complex technique and Vector Red substrate (Vector Laboratories). Smooth muscle cells were identified by immunostaining with an alkaline-phosphatase-conjugated monoclonal antibody to α-smooth muscle actin (clone 1A4, Sigma, St. Louis, MO). Sections were counterstained with hematoxylin.

2.3 Tissue preparation reverse transcription-polymerase chain reaction

At death, mice were perfused with 0.9% NaCl solution and the femoral artery was quickly excised. Total RNA was prepared with the use of RNazol reagent (TEL-TEST, INC., Friendswood, TX). Reverse transcription was performed with random hexamer primers and MMLV reverse transcriptase (ReverTraAce-α, TOYOBO, Osaka). PCR primers were as follows: α-smooth muscle actin, 5′-GAGAAGCCCAGCCAGTCG-3′ and 5′-CTCTTGCTCTGGGCTTCA-3′; glyceraldehydes-3-phosphate dehydrogenase (GAPDH), 5′-ACCACAGTCCATGCCATCAC-3′ and 5′-TCCAC CACCCTGTTGCTGTA-3′. PCR reactions were carried out 30 cycles of 45 seconds of denaturation at 94°C, 45 seconds of annealing at 60°C, and 2 minutes of extension at 72°C followed by 10 minutes of final extension.

2.4 Cell culture

Total bone marrow cells were isolated from wild-type mice as described. 4×10^6 cells were cultured in a well of 24-well dish in Dulbeccos's modified eagle medium (Sigma) containing 10% FBS, 10 ng/ml PDGF-BB, 10 ng/ml basic FGF. Cell suspensions were treated with ACK lysing buffer (0.155 M ammonium chloride, 0.1 M disodium EDTA and 0.01 M potassium bicarbonate) to lyse erythrocytes. After washing, cells were suspended in serum-free medium (X-vivo 20, BioWhittaker/Takara, Tokyo) and cultured in a fibronectin-coated 24-well dish. For immunocytochemistry, cells were fixed in 4% paraformaldehyde. After permeabilized with 0.5% NP40 in PBS, cells were stained with an alkaline-phosphatase-conjugated monoclonal antibody to α-smooth muscle actin (clone 1A4, Sigma, St. Louis, MO) and Vector Red substrate (Vector Laboratories).

2.5 Statistical analysis

All values are expressed as mean $\pm$ SEM. The means were compared by the unpaired Student's t-test. A value of $P < 0.05$ was considered statistically significant.

3 Results

3.1 Time course of neointimal hyperplasia

A large wire was inserted into the femoral artery, causing complete endothelial denudation and marked enlargement of lumen with acute onset of

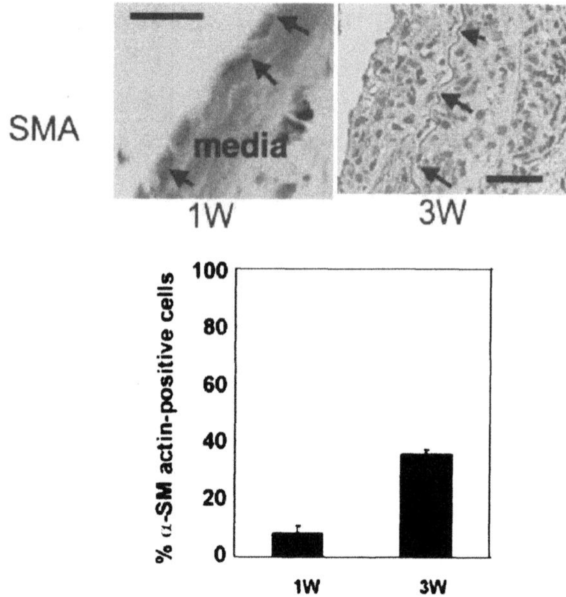

Fig. 1. Temporal and spatial characterization of cellular constituents during neo-intima hyperplasia development. SMA positive cells gradually increased. SMA-positive cells were counted and expressed as proportion to the total number of the cells in the vessel wall. Data are reported as mean ± S.E.M. n = 3 for each time point. Arrows indicate internal elastic lamina. Bar, 20 μm.

medial SMCs apoptosis. Cellular constituents of the arterial wall after wire-mediated injury was examined by RT-PCR using RNA obtained from total homogenate of the vessel wall. Marked downregulation of α-smooth muscle actin (α-SMA) expression was observed at one week. α-SMA expression gradually increased at two weeks and reached to that of uninjured artery at 4 and 6 weeks (Date not shown). Cellular constituents of the arterial wall were also evaluated by immunohistochemistry. At one week, small neo-intima was found on the luminal side of the injured artery. Most of the neointimal cells expressed CD45, a marker for hematopoietic cells, but not α-SMA (Figs. 1, 2). At three weeks, large neointima had grown on the luminal side. A few CD45-positive cells were detected, particularly in the luminal side of the neointima. There were some α-SMA-positive cells.

In uninujred arteries, the endothelium lined at luminal side of the internal elastic lamina. At two hours after injury, the artery remained dilated with a thin media containing very few cells. Fibrin deposition and platelets accumulation were observed on the denuded luminal side.

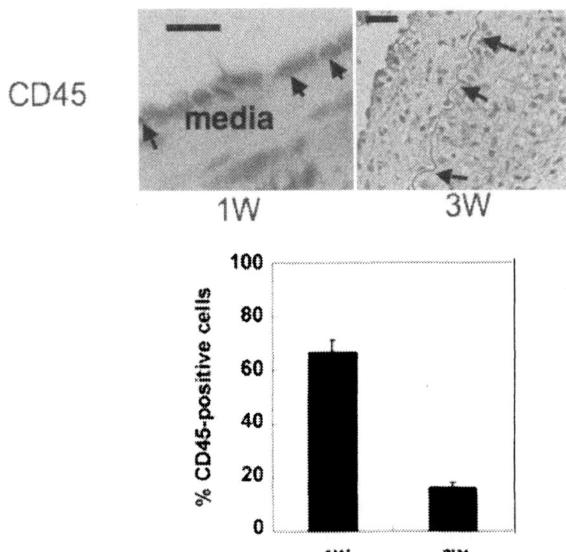

Fig. 2. CD45 positive cells gradually decreased. CD45-positive cells were counted and expressed as proportion to the total number of the cells in the vessel wall. Data are reported as mean ± S.E.M. n = 3 for each time point. Arrows indicate internal elastic lamina. Bar, 20 μm.

3.2 Cell culture

Total bone marrow cells were plated on a plastic dish in the presence of 10% serum. At four days, floating cells were washed. PDGF-BB (10 ng/ml) was added to the adherent cells. Immunocytochemistry (8 days) and RT-PCR (20 days) reveled that those cells expressed α smooth muscle actin (α-SMA). In the presence of PDGF-BB (10 ng/ml) and basic FGF (10 ng/ml), those adherent cells differentiated into smooth muscle-like cells, which expressed α-SMA (Fig. 3).

4 Discussion

We investigated the cellular constituents spatially and temporally during development of neointimal hyperplasia after mechanical vascular injury. This injury causes severe damage characterized by complete endothelial denudation and massive apoptosis of medial cells. As early as at two hours after injury, the denuded lumen was coated with deposition of fibrin with aggregated platelets. At one week, CD45-positive, α-SMA-negative

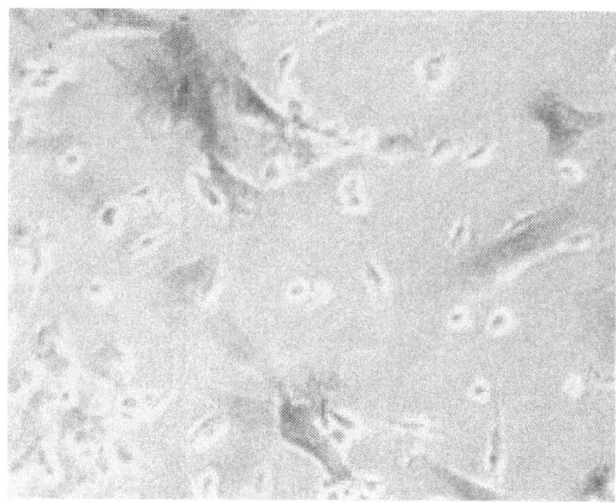

Fig. 3. Contribution of bone marrow-derived cells to neointimal formation. Bone marrow cells differentiated into smooth muscle-like cells, which expressed α-SMA. (8 days after cell culture).

hematopoietic cells were homing at the luminal side as determined by immunocytochemisty and scanning electron microscope. Following accumulation of hematopoietic cells, α-SMA positive neointima hyperplasia developed. These findings suggest that circulating blood cells may contribute to α-SMA positive SMC-like cells in neointima. This hypothesis was supported by the observations that bone marrow cells and circulating blood cells could differentiate into α-SMA-positive cells *in vitro* and *in vivo*.

Coronary angioplasty causes vessel wall injury and induces SMCs proliferation with subsequent abundant production of extracellular matrix. Angioplasty denudes endothelium completely and mechanically dilates atherosclerotic lesions with a tear in the luminal surface (Sata 2003). Therefore, neointima formation appears to be similar to the healing process in response to vascular injuries. In addition to the conventional assumption that damaged tissues are repaired by individual parenchymal cells, an accumulating body of evidence indicates that there exist somatic stem cells that are mobilized to remote organs, differentiate into required lineages and participate in organ repair and regeneration (Sata M 2000, Rafii S 2003, McKay R 2000, Hill JM 2003) Bone marrow might be an additional source of vascular cells that contribute to repair and remodeling of vessel wall. Consistent with this notion, an analysis of sex-mismatched bone marrow transplant subjects revealed that SMCs throughout the atherosclerotic vessel wall can derive from donor bone marrow (Caplice NM 2003). Of interest is a finding that recruitment of bone marrow-derived SMCs was more extensive in diseased compared with undiseased segments.

It still remained to be elucidated what kind of stimuli promote differentiation of circulating progenitors into α-actin positive cells. At very early stage after injury, the denudated vessel wall was quickly coated with fibrin and platelets. Our *in vitro* experiment showed that fibronectin, basic FGF, and PDGF-BB are essential for differentiation of peripheral mononuclear cells into α-actin positive cells. Fibronectin binds to fibrin and aggregated platelets secret PDGF. It may be plausible that endothelial injury and subsequent deposition of platelets and fibrin may provide optimal conditions for homing and differentiation of circulating smooth muscle progenitors.

In summary, our results suggest that overstretching and endothelial denudation cause rapid accumulation of fibrin and platelets, which may favor homing and differentiation of circulating progenitors. Our findings may provide further insights into the mechanism of vascular repair and lesion formation after severe mechanical injury.

5 Conclusion

Our study suggest that early accumulation of hematopoietic cells may play a role in the pathogenesis of smooth muscle cells hyperplasia under certain circumstances.

References

Caplice NM, Bunch TJ, Stalboerger PG, Wang S, Simpler D, Miller DV, Russell SJ, Litzow MR, Edwards WD et al. (2003) Smooth muscle cells in human coronary atherosclerosis can originate from cells administered at marrow transplantation. Proc Natl Acad Sci U S A 100:4754–4759.

Hill JM, Zalos G, Halcox JP, Schenke WH, Waclawiw MA, Quyyumi AA, Finkle T (2003) Circulating endothelial progenitor cells, vascular function, and cardiovascular risk. N Engl J Med 348:593–600.

Kearney M, Pieczek A, Haley L, Losordo DW, Andres V, Schainfeld R, Rosenfield K, Isner JM (1997). Histopathology of in-stent restenosis in patients with peripheral artery disease. Circulation 95:1998–2002.

Korbling M, Katz RL, Khanna A, Ruifrok AC, Rondon G, Albitar M, Champlin RE, Estrov Z (2002) Hepatocytes and epithelial cells of donor origin in recipients of peripheral-blood stem cells. N Engl J Med 346:738–746.

McKay R (2000) Stem cells-hype and hope. Nature 406:361–364.

Nobuyoshi M, Kimura T, Nosaka H, Mioka S, Ueno K, Yokoi H, Hamasaki N, Horiuchi H, Ohishi H (1988) Restenosis after successful percutaneous transluminal coronary angioplasty: serial angiographic follow-up of 229 patients. J Am Coll Cardiol 12:616–623.

Nobuyoshi M, Kimura T, Ohishi H, Horiuchi H, Nosaka H, Hamasaki N, Yokoi H, Kim K et al. (1991) Restenosis after percutaneous transluminal coronary angioplasty: pathologic observations in 20 patients. J Am Coll Cardiol 17:433–439.

Rafii S and Lyden D (2003) Therapeutic stem and progenitor cell transplantation for organ vascularization and regeneration. Nat Med 9:702–712.

Saiura A, Sata M, Hirata Y, Nagai R, Makuuchi M (2001) Circulating smooth muscle progenitor cells contribute to atherosclerosis. Nat Med 7:382–383.

Sata M (2000) Circulating vascular progenitor cells contribute to vascular repair, remodeling, and lesion formation. Trends Cardiovasc Med 13:249–253.

Sata M, Maejima Y, Adachi F, Fukino K, Saiura A, Sugiura S, Aoyagi T, Imai Y, Kurihara H, Kimura K, Omata M, Makuuchi M, Hirata Y, Nagai R (2000) A mouse model of vascular injury that induces rapid onset of medial cell apoptosis followed by reproducible neointimal hyperplasia. J Mol Cell Cardiol 32:2097–2104.

Sata M, Saiura A, Kunisato A, Tojo A, Okada S, Tokuhisa T, Hirai H, Makuuchi M, Hirata Y, Nagai R et al. (2002) Hematopoietic stem cells differentiate into vascular cells that participate in the pathogenesis of atherosclerosis. Nat Med 8:403–409.

Sata M (2003) Circulating vascular progenitor cells contribute to vascular repair, remodeling, and lesion formation. Trends Cardiovasc Med 13:249–253.

TNF-α mobilizes bone marrow derived cells to vascular wall, resulting in neointima formation through its inflammatory effects

Makoto Shoji[1], Hiroshi Suzuki[1], Taro Kusuyama[1], Yasutoshi Omori[1], Teruko Soda[1], Fumiyoshi Tsunoda[1], Takatoshi Sato[1], Shinji Koba[1], Eiichi Geshi[1], Takashi Katagiri[1], Seiji Shioda[2]

[1]Third Department of Internal Medicine and [2]First Department of Anatomy, Showa University School of Medicine, 1-5-8 Hatanodai, Shinagawa-ku, Tokyo 142-8555, Japan

Summary. Background: Recent studies suggest that bone marrow cells contribute to neointimal formation after vascular injury. However, the relationship between the inflammatory reactions and bone marrow cell invasion has not been clarified. Method and Results: We insert a large wire (0.38 mm in a diameter) into the femoral arteries of 6–8 week-old male balb/c (WT) and TNF-α Knockout (KO) mice. In imunohistochmistry using CD34 at 1 week, positive cells possibly containing bone marrow derived cells, were hardly observed in KO, but some were observed in WT in neointima. At 4 weeks, CD45 positive cells were rarely seen, and α-smooth muscle actin positive cells were main component of thickened neointima in both groups. In morphometric analysis at 4 weeks after the injury, developed neointimal area was smaller in KO. Furthermore, re-endothelialization appeared earlier in KO than WT. Conclusion: TNF-α is involved in neointimal formation after vascular injury, possible through its inflammatory effects to induce bone marrow cells.

Key words. TNF-α, bone marrow derived cells, arterial remodeling, CD34

1 Introduction

For treatment of re-stenosis after percutaneus coronary intervention (PCI), it is very important to clarify the detail mechanism of process of neointimal hyperplasia. Ross et al. (Ross 1993) indicated that smooth muscle cells in the neointima after PCI had been derived from media at injured artery. But recent studies suggest that bone marrow cells contribute to neointimal formation after vascular injury (Saiura 2001). We have been reported that bone marrow cells could give rise to vascular progenitor cells that potentially contribute to pathological remodeling in models of post-PCI restenosis (Sata 2000, 2002, 2003). In many factors to relate with bone marrow cells mobilization, local inflammation induced by cytokines is possible to derive bone marrow cells to vascular wall, resulting thickened neointima.

Inflammatory cytokine, TNF-α is mainly produced by activated monocytes and macrophages that elicit cytotoxic activity and cell activation in various cell types by signal transduction. TNF-α itself modulated neointimal hyperplasia induced by low shear stress (Rectenwalds 2000). However, the relationship between the inflammatory reactions of TNF-α and bone marrow cell invasion has not been clarified.

Here we performed vascular injury model using TNF-α knockout mice (KO) to investigate the involvement of inflammation on bone marrow cells mobilization in the process of neointimal formation.

2 Method

2.1 Animal experimental protocol

Adult male 16- to 24-week-old inbred wild-type mice (balb/c) or TNF-α KO mice (balb/c background) (Taniguchi 1997) weighing between 25 and 35 g were used. For all surgical procedures, the mice were anesthetized. Transluminal mechanical injury of the femoral artery was induced by insertion of a large wire (0.38 mm in diameter) as previously described (Shoji 2004, Sata 2000). The mice were euthanized by intraperitoneal administration of an overdose of Nembutal at 1 and 4 weeks after the injury. At death, the mice were perfused with 0.9% NaCl solution followed by perfusion fixation with 4% paraformaldehyde in PBS (pH 7.4). The femoral artery was carefully excised, further fixed in 4% paraformaldehyde overnight, and embedded in paraffin. Cross-sections (5 μm) were stained with hematoxylin and eosin.

2.2 Immunohistochemistry

Paraffin-embedded sections (5 μm) were deparaffinized, blocked with 0.5% goat serum, and incubated with an anti-mouse CD34 antibody (clone

H-140, Santa Cruz) or anti-mouse CD45 antibody (clone 30-F11, BD Pharmingen). Antibody distribution was visualized by the avidin-biotin complex technique and Vector Red substrate (Vector Laboratories). Smooth muscle cells were identified by immunostaining with monoclonal antibody to α-smooth muscle actin (α-SMA) (clone 1A4, Sigma). Sections were counterstained with hematoxylin.

2.3 Cell culture

Total bone marrow cells were isolated from WT or TNF-α KO mice as described. Cells of 4×10^6 were cultured in a well of 24-well dish in Dulbeccos's modified eagle medium (Sigma) containing 10% FBS, 10 ng/ml PDGF-BB, 10 ng/ml basic FGF.

For immunocytochemistry, cells were fixed in 4% paraformaldehyde. After permeabilized with 0.5% NP40 in PBS, cells were stained with an alkaline-phosphatase-conjugated monoclonal antibody to α-SMA (clone 1A4, Sigma) and Vector Red substrate (Vector Laboratories).

2.4 Statistical analysis

All values are expressed as mean $\pm$ SEM. The means were compared by the unpaired Student's t-test. A value of $P < 0.05$ was considered statistically significant.

3 Results

3.1 Histochemical and immunohistochemical analysis

In time course, accumulation of CD45 positive cells at the luminal side of thin neointima peaked at 1 week in both groups. At 4 weeks, CD45 positive cells were rarely seen, and α-SMA positive cells were main component of thickened neointima. In morphometric analysis at 4 weeks after the injury, developed neointimal area was smaller in KO (intima/media ratio: 2.99 ± 0.24 versus 1.52 ± 0.15, $P < 0.05$) (Fig. 1), and the number of inflammatory cells such as neutrophils, macrophages and apoptotic cells in neointima were much less in KO than in wild type. Furthermore, re-endothelialization appeared earlier in KO than WT (Date not shown). In imunohistochmistry using CD34 at 1 week, positive cells possibly containing bone marrow derived cells, were hardly observed in KO, but some were

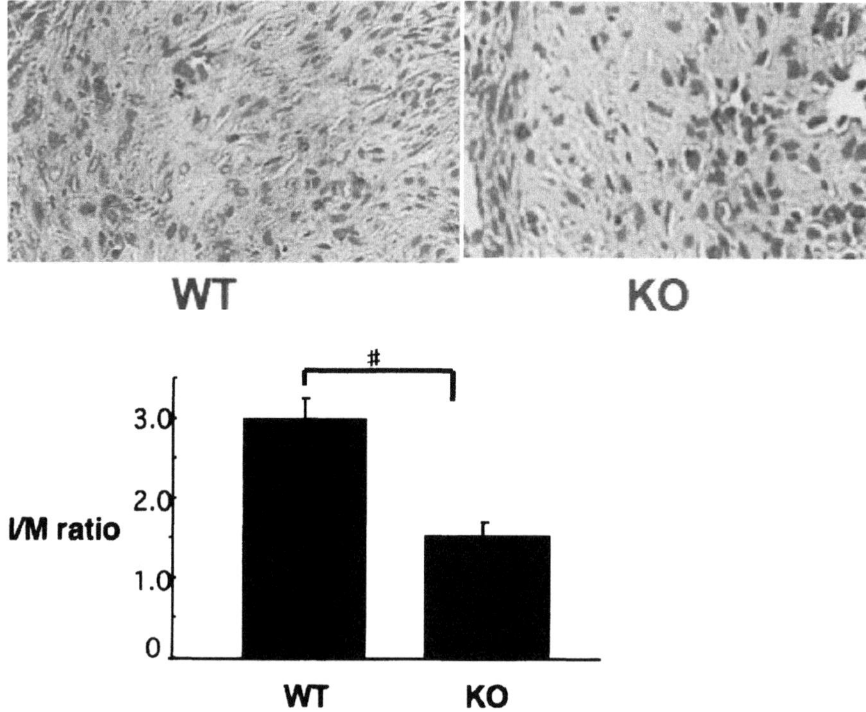

Fig. 1. Neointimal hyperplasia was inhibited in TNF-α knockout mice. Injured arteries were embedded in paraffin and stained with hematoxyline and eosin. Graph demonstrates development of the neointima after vascular injury. Data are reported as mean ± S.E.M.

observed in WT in neointima (Fig. 2). At 4 weeks. CD34 positive cells were not observed in both groups.

3.2 Cell culture

Total bone marrow cells which were plated on a plastic dish in the presence of 10% serum. At 4 days, floating cells were washed and PDGF-BB (10 ng/ml) was added to the adherent cells. In the presence of PDGF-BB (10 ng/ml) and basic FGF (10 ng/ml), those adherent cells differentiated into smooth muscle-like cells, expressing α-SMA. Immunocytochemistry reveled that those cells expressed α-SMA, which was not expressed in bone marrow cells before culture. In KO group, α-SMA positive cells tend to be less than in wild type group (Fig. 3).

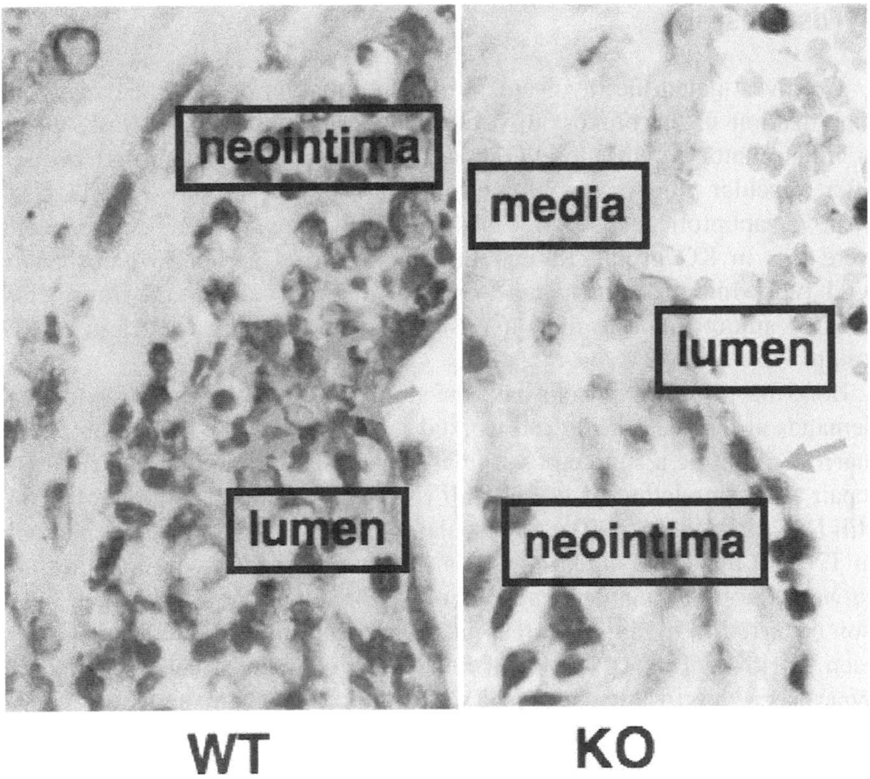

Fig. 2. Bone marrow derived cells were less in TNF-α knockout mice. Cross-sections were performed immunohistochemistry of CD34 antibody. Arrow heads indicated CD34 positive cells.

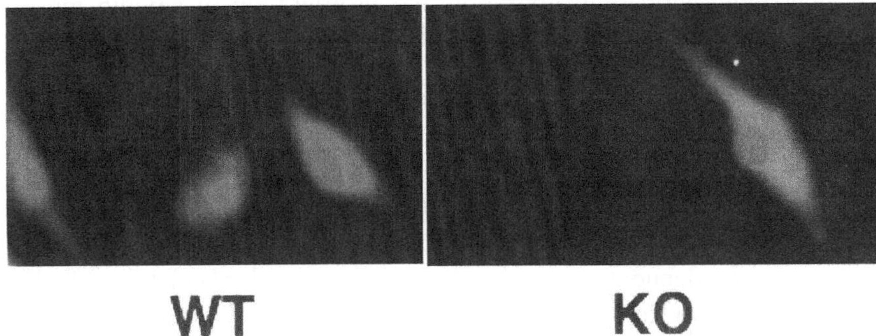

Fig. 3. Differentiation of bone marrow cells into α-actin positive cells. In TNF-α knockout mice, α-SMA positive cells tend to be less than in wild type mice.

4 Discussion

We investigated the involvement of inflammation on bone marrow cells mobilization in the process of neointimal formation using TNF-α, which is inflammatory cytokine, KO mice. In vivo study, neointimal portion after vascular injury was smaller in TNF-α KO group. The TUNEL positive, apoptotic cells and CD34 positive, bone marrow derived cells were less in KO group. Re-endothelium occurred earlier in KO than in wild type. In vitro study, bone marrow derived cells could transdifferentiated smooth muscle marker positive cells, and they were less in KO group.

Bone marrow derived cells have the ability of transdifferentiation to what demands at injured portion and worked repair (Sata 2003). Therefore, bone marrow might be a source of vascular cells in neointima that contribute to repair and remodeling of vessel wall (McKay R 2000, Caplice NM 2003, Hill JM 2003, Rafii S 2003). At vascular injury, inflammatory cytokine such as TNF-α, may be a signal at needs for repair. However, the relationship between the inflammatory reactions of TNF-α and bone marrow cell invasion occurred in the injured area, inducing neointimal proliferation has not been clarified. TNF-α itself had been known to be affected neointimal hyperplasia due to low shear stress by multiple mechanisms (Rectenwald JM 2000). In the present study, apoptosis and inflammatory reaction occurred in the vascular wall after vascular injury in both WT and TNF-α KO mice, however, we observed much less apoptotic and inflammatory cells in TNF-α KO mice. Furthermore, we observed more CD34 positive cells in more inflammatory cells accumulated portion, especially in WT mice than KO mice. Inflammatory cell invasion may be the inducer to mobilize bone marrow derived cells. Our *in vitro* experiment showed that TNF-α modulated differentiation of bone marrow cells into α-actin positive cells. TNF-α may contribute activation, migration and proliferation of smooth muscle cells at injured artery, partly through the inhibiting mobilization of bone-marrow cells (Rectenwald JM 2000).

It still remained to be elucidated what kind of stimuli after the activation of TNF-α promote differentiation of bone marrow derived progenitors into α-actin positive cells. TNF-α induced expression of biologically active molecules, such as ICAM-1 that may accentuate the fibroproliferation response to injury (Oguro 2002, Hui 2004 Shibata 2005). At very early stage after injury, the denudated vessel wall was coated with platelets and leukocytes (Shoji 2004). Injured artery secreted ICAM-1 and subsequent aggregated monocytes and leukocytes. It may be plausible that endothelial injury and subsequent deposition of fibrin and leukocytes may provide optimal conditions for homing and differentiation of bone marrow derived smooth muscle progenitor cells. ICAM-1 activation induced by TNF-α may be involved in the process.

5 Conclusion

TNF-α is involved in neointimal formation after vascular injury, possible through its inflammatory effects to induce bone marrow cells.

References

Caplice NM, Bunch TJ, Stalboerger PG, Wang S, Simpler D, Miller DV, Russell SJ, Litzow MR, Edwards WD (2003) Smooth muscle cells in human coronary atherosclerosis can originate from cells administered at marrow transplantation. Proc Natl Acad Sci U S A 100:4754–4759.

Hill JM, Zalos G, Halcox JP, Schenke WH, Waclawiw MA, Quyyumi AA, Finkle T (2003) Circulating endothelial progenitor cells, vascular function, and cardiovascular risk. N Engl J Med 348:593–600.

Hui Y, Min L, Hong C, Shaoryu Y, Rongxin Z, Qizhi Y, Changyi C (2004) Expression and Regulation of Neuropilins and VEGF Receptors by TNF-α in Human Endothelial Cells. Journal of Surgical Research 122:249–255.

McKay R (2000) Stem cells-hype and hope. Nature 406:361–364.

Oguro T, Takahashi Y, Takahashi Y, Ashino T, Takaki A, Shioda S, Horai R, Asano M, Sekikawa K, Iwakura Y, Yoshida T (2002) Involvement of tumor necrosis factor α, rather than interleukin-1α/β or nitric oxides in the heme oxygenase-1 gene expression by lipopolysaccharide in the mouse liver. FEBS Letters 515:63–66.

Rafii S and Lyden D (2003) Therapeutic stem and progenitor cell transplantation for organ vascularization and regeneration. Nat Med 9:702–712.

Rectenwald JE, Moldawer LL, Huber TS, Seeger JM, Ozaki CK (2000) Direct evidence for cytokine involvement in neointimal hyperplasia 102(14): 1697–1702.

Ross R (1993) the pathogenesis of atherosclerosis:a perspective for the 1990s.

Saiura A, Sata M, Hirata Y, Nagai R, Makuuchi M (2001) Circulating smooth muscle progenitor cells contribute to atherosclerosis. Nat Med 7:382–383.

Sata M (2000) Circulating vascular progenitor cells contribute to vascular repair, remodeling, and lesion formation. Trends Cardiovasc Med 13:249–253.

Sata M, Maejima Y, Adachi F, Fukino K, Saiura A, Sugiura S, Aoyagi T, Imai Y, Kurihara H, Kimura K, Omata M, Makuuchi M, Hirata Y, Nagai R (2000) A mouse model of vascular injury that induces rapid onset of medial cell apoptosis followed by reproducible neointimal hyperplasia. J Mol Cell Cardiol;32:2097–2104.

Sata M, Saiura A, Kunisato A, Tojo A, Okada S, Tokuhisa T, Hirai H, Makuuchi M, Hirata Y, Nagai R (2002) Hematopoietic stem cells differentiate into vascular cells that participate in the pathogenesis of atherosclerosis. Nat Med 8:403–409.

Sata M (2003) Circulating vascular progenitor cells contribute to vascular repair, remodeling, and lesion formation. Trends Cardiovasc Med 13:249–253.

Shibata M, Sueki H, Suzuki H, Watanabe H, Ohtaki H, Shioda S, Nakanishi-Ueda T, Yasuhara H, Sekikawa K, Iijima (2005) Impaired Contact Hypersensitivity Reaction and Reduced Production of Vascular Endothelial Growth Factor in Tumor Necrosis Factor-α Gene–Deficient Mice. The Journal of Dermatology 32:523–533.

Shoji M, Sata M, Fukuda D, Tahaka K, Sato T, Iso Y, Shibata M, Suzuki H, Koba S, Geshi E, Katagiri T (2004) Temporal and spatial characterization of cellular constituents during neointimal hyperplasia after vascular injury: Potential contribution of bone marrow derived progenitors to arterial remodeling Cardiovascular Pathology 13:306–312.

Sugano M, Tsuchida K, Makino N (2004) Intramuscular gene transfer of soluble tumor necrosis factor-alpha receptor 1 activates vascular endothelial growth factor receptor and accelerates angiogenesis in a rat model of hindlimb ischemia. Circulation 109(6):797–802.

Taniguchi T, Takata M, Ikeda A, Momotani E, Sekikawa K (1997) Failure of Germinal Center Formation and Impairment of Response to Endotoxin in Tumor Necrosis Factor α-Deficient Mice Lab Invest 77:647–658.

Angiogenesis induced by adhesion between polymorphonuclear leukocyte and endothelial cell via intercellular adhesion molecule-1

Masako Yasuda[1], Masayuki Ohbayashi[1], Shunichi Shimizu[2], Toshinori Yamamoto[1]

[1]Department of Clinical Pharmacy, and [2]Pathophysiology Pharmaceutical Sciences of Showa University, 1-5-8, Hatanodai, Shinagawa-ku, Tokyo 142-8555, Japan

Summary. We demonstrate that adhesion between polymorphonuclear leukocyte (PMN) and endothelial cells (ECs) is concerned with induction of angiogenesis of ECs. For the tube formation assay, ECs obtained from bovine thoracic aorta (BAECs) grown on a layer of collagen type I were used. Addition of PMNs treated with N-formyl-methionyl-leucyl-phenylalanine (FMLP), a selective activator of PMN induced angiogenesis. The angiogenesis was blocked by monoclonal antibodies against E-selectin and intercellular adhesion molecule-1 (ICAM-1) which inhibit the adhesion between PMN and EC. Ets-1, which stimulates metalloproteinase gene transcription or integrin β_3, has a key role in angiogenesis. Addition of activated PMNs to ECs stimulated the angiogenesis and Ets-1 expression. Both the angiogenesis and the Ets-1 expression induced by PMNs were reduced by ets-1 antisense oligonucleotide. On the other hand, PMN-induced Ets-1 expression was reduced by a monoclonal antibody against ICAM-1 but not E-selectin despite the inhibition of PMN-induced angiogenesis by both antibodies. The enhancement of angiogenesis by FMLP-treated PMNs was blocked by catalase, a scavenging enzyme of H_2O_2, but not by superoxide dismutase (SOD). Interestingly, the stimulation of angiogenesis by H_2O_2 without PMNs was inhibited by anti E-selectin antibody but not anti ICAM-1. ICAM-1 stimulation occurred by ICAM-1 cross-linking enhanced angiogenesis. These findings indicated that PMN adhesion was related with the induction of angiogenesis, and ICAM-1 in endothelial cells acted as a signaling receptor to induce Ets-1 expression, whereas E-selectin seemed to function in the formation of tube-like structures in vascular endothelial cell cultures.

84

Key words. Angiogenesis, polymorphonuclear leukocyte, ICAM-1, Ets-1, H_2O_2

1 Introduction

Angiogenesis, the formation of new blood vessels, occurs under various physiological conditions (Folkman 1995). Especially in inflammatory diseases such as wound healing, chronic inflammation, solid tumor formation, and diabetic retinopathy, it has been suggested that angiogenesis is involved in the maintenance of the inflammatory state by transporting inflammatory cells to the site of inflammation and supplying nutrients and oxygen to the inflamed tissue (Jackson et al. 1997). In fact, rheumatoid arthritis and the skin of psoriatic disease, the proliferating tissue contains an abundance of inflammatory cells, angiogenic blood vessels and inflammatory mediators (Koch et al. 1992, Koch et al. 1994). Furthermore, it is reported that activated monocytes and macrophages are able to produce growth factors and cytokines which regulate angiogenesis (Sunderkotter et al. 1994, Koch et al. 1986). However, the role of neutrophils, another type of inflammatory cells in angiogenesis has not been fully evaluated. The recruitment of PMNs is believed to be one of the important mechanisms in the pathophysiology of various inflammatory diseases (Vissers et al. 1985).

PMNs activated during inflammation adhere to ECs (Babior et al. 2000, Weissmann et al. 1980). The adherence of PMNs to ECs is mediated by adhesion molecules such as E-selectin and ICAM-1 expressed in endothelial cells (Gasic et al. 1991, Del Zoppo 1997). Recently, adhesion molecules have been reported to act as the signaling receptors that mediate changes in intracellular Ca^{2+} concentration (Lorenzon et al. 1998) and tyrosine phosphorylation (Durieu-Trautmann et al. 1994). Therefore, we investigated the effect of the adhesion molecules on the angiogenesis.

Ets-1 is a transcription factor that regulates the gene expression of proteases such as urokinase-type plasminogen activator (u-PA), matrix metalloproteinase (MMP)-1, MMP-3, and MMP-9 (Sato 1998). Many studies have shown that Ets-1 mediates angiogenesis. Iwasaka et al. (1996) reported that vascular endothelial growth factor (VEGF) and basic fibroblast growth factor (bFGF) induce Ets-1 expression and Ets-1 stimulates angiogenesis.

Previously, we reported that low concentration of H_2O_2 induced angiogenesis mediated by ets-1 expression (Yasuda et al. 1999). Moreover, a non toxic concentration of ROS has been shown to stimulate cell growth and increase the transcription factors, such as NF-κB and AP-1 in the endothelial cells (Barchowsky et al. 1995). Thus, it is thought that ROS is one of the physiological regulators for cell functions (Irani 2000). Therefore, it is possible that the signal transduction from adhesion molecules induces Ets-1 mediated by H_2O_2 and then stimulates angiogenesis.

We report that the angiogenesis induced by PMN adhesion via ICAM-1 regulated by the transcriptional factor ets-1, and H_2O_2 is related with the regulation of the angiogenesis.

2 Materials and methods

Cell—Bovine aortic endothelial cells (BAECs) were obtained from the aorta of Japanese cattle. PMNs were collected from male Wistar rats (6–8 weeks old). Human umbilical vein endothelial cells (HUVEC) at 5–10 passages were used for experiments. *ICAM-1 cross-linking*—HUVECs were incubated with 1 µg/mL murine anti-human ICAM-1 ligation antibody for 30 min. For the cross-linking study, the anti-human ICAM-1 ligation antibody which recognize 46 to 160 amino acid domain, clone 28 was used (BD Transduction Laboratories). After incubation, the cells were washed with PBS, and were treated with 10 µg/mL goat IgG (H + L) against murine IgG. *In vitro angiogenesis*—Tube formation was measured using the three-dimensional culture method. The angiogenesis of BAECs was carried out on re-constituted collagen type I gel. When the BAECs culture reached confluent, various concentrations of PMNs with or without Met-Leu-Phe (FMLP) (1 µM), a selective stimulant of PMN, and incubated for 3 days. For angiogenesis of HUVECs, the cells were added into the Matrigel-coated 48-well plates and cultured for 24 hrs after ICAM-1 stimulation. Tube-like structures formed by ECs were quantified by measuring the total additive length of all cellular structures including all branches, using a computer-assisted image analyzer. *Measurement of mRNA expression*—The ets-1 mRNA expression was measured by Northern blotting method. The signal intensity was quantified with an imaging analyzer and indicated as the ratio of ets-1/GAPDH signal intensity.

3 Results and discussion

Under control conditions, BAECs grew to confluent monolayers in a cobblestone pattern on the surface of collagen gels (Fig. 1A) (Yasuda et al. 2002). After addition of PMNs, BAECs formed a network of branching cellular cords beneath the surface monolayer, suggesting the induction of angiogenesis (Fig. 1B) (Yasuda et al. 2002). The enhancement of angiogenesis was induced by concentration-dependent manner PMN (Yasuda et al.

86

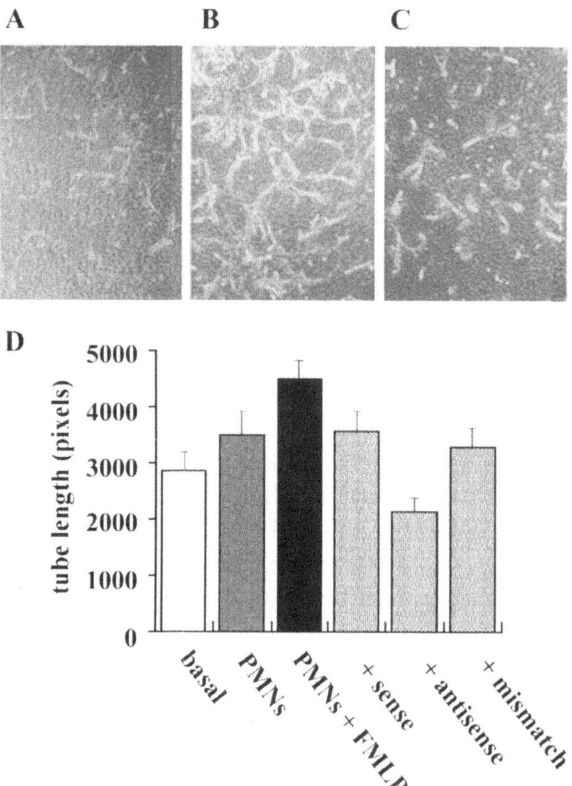

Fig. 1. Effects of ets-1 antisense oligonucleotide on PMN-induced angiogenesis in BAECs. Endothelial cells were cultured on collagen gel in 24-well plates to confluence, and then minimum essential medium (MEM) containing 0.1% FBS and 1×10^5 PMNs/ml stimulated with or without $1\,\mu$M FMLP were added to the cells and incubated for 72 h. *ets*-1 sense, antisense, or mismatch oligonucleotide (all at $3\,\mu$M) was added to the BAECs 6 h before addition of PMNs. The sequences of the oligonucleotides of *ets*-1 were as follows: ATG AAG GCG GCC GTC GAT CT (sense), AGA TCG ACG GCC GCC TTC AT (antisense), and ATG CAC AGC TCC GCC AGG TT (mismatch). The cultures were fixed with 0.25% glutaraldehyde and photographed (original magnification ×100). Photomicrographs show control (A), treatment with activated PMNs (B), and effects of ets-1 antisense oligonucleotide on activated PMN-induced angiogenesis (C). The tube-like structures formed were quantified by measuring the total additive length of all cellular structures including all branches with a computer-assisted image analyzer (D). Results are expressed as the means $\pm$ SE of 3 experiments. $^{\dagger}P < 0.05$ vs. basal; $*P < 0.05$ vs. PMNs with FMLP. "From Am J Physiol Cell Physiol 282 (2002), with permission."

2000) and the angiogenesis was significantly increased by simultaneous treatment with 1 μM FMLP (Fig. 1D) (Yasuda et al. 2002). However, addition of FMLP alone or the supernatant from PMNs to BAECs did not induce any morphological changes including angiogenesis.

PMNs adhere to endothelial cells via adhesion molecules such as ICAM-1 and E-selectin. Adhesion molecules were initially thought to function only in cell adhesion between vascular endothelial cells and leukocytes (Del Maschio et al. 1996, Lo et al. 1992). However, adhesion of PMNs to endothelial cells was reported recently to trigger various physiological changes including an increase in intracellular Ca^{2+} concentration and activation of transcription factor nuclear factor-κB (Barchowsky et al. 1995, Lorenzon et al. 1998). Anti-ICAM-1 and anti-E-selectin antibodies, which inhibited adhesion between PMNs, prevented PMN-induced angiogenesis by endothelial cells (Fig. 2) (Yasuda et al. 2000). Thus both ICAM-1 and E-selectin seem to be essential factors for PMN-induced angiogenesis.

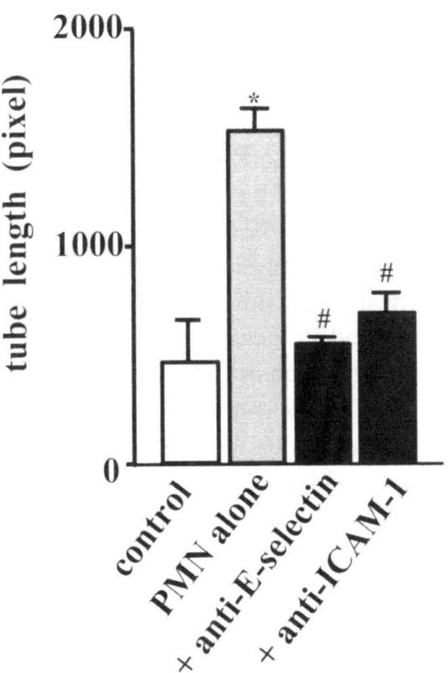

Fig. 2. Effects of anti-E-selectin and anti-ICAM- antibodies on PMN-induced angiogenesis. BAECs were preincubated with or without anti-E-selectin (5 μg/mL) or anti-ICAM- (5 μg/mL) monoclonal antibody for 30 min. FMLP (1 μM)-treated or -untreated PMN was then added to BAECs and incubated for 3 days. Results are expressed as the means ± SE of 3 experiments with triplicate determinations in each assay. *P < 0.05 vs. BAEC control, #P < 0.05 vs. FMLP-treated PMNs. "From Am J Physiol Cell Physiol 282 (2002), with permission."

The relation of a transcription factor, ets-1 which plays an important role of angiogenesis regulation on PMN-induced angiogenesis was investigated. Ets-1 is one of the important transcription factors which regulate angiogenesis. The ets-1 induces matrix metalloproteinases genes such as matrix metalloproteinase (MMP)-1, MMP-3, MMP-9, urokinase-type plasminogen activator, integrin β_3 associated with angiogenesis-related molecules (Oda et al. 1999). The PMN-induced angiogenesis was attenuated by the pretreatment of ets-1 antisense but not sense or mismatch oligonucleotide (Fig. 1C and D) (Yasuda et al. 2002).

The ets-1 mRNA expression increased from 3 to 6 hrs after the addition of PMN to the endothelial cells (Yasuda et al. 2002). These results suggested that PMN-induced angiogenesis was promoted by ets-1. Interestingly, PMN-induced increase of ets-1 mRNA expression was inhibited by anti-ICAM-1 antibody but not by anti-E-selectin antibody although both the antibodies of ICAM-1 and E-selectin blocked PMN-induced angiogenesis (Fig. 3) (Yasuda et al. 2002). ICAM-1 but not E-selectin might act as a signaling receptor for the induction of Ets-1.

Activated PMNs have been shown to release reactive oxygen species (ROS) including H_2O_2 (Hoffstein et al. 1985, Kopprasch et al. 1995). We previously reported that H_2O_2 stimulates angiogenesis through the induction of Ets-1 (Yasuda et al. 1999). Also PMN-stimulated angiogenesis and ets-1 mRNA expression were inhibited by catalase but not by SOD (Yasuda et al. 2000). Thus H_2O_2 released from PMNs seems to be involved in the stimulation of angiogenesis through the induction of Ets-1 expression. Interestingly, H_2O_2-induced angiogenesis was inhibited by anti-E-selectin antibody but not by anti-ICAM-1 antibody (Yasuda et al. 2002). Nguyen et al. (1993) previously reported that formation of tube-like structures by BAEC cultured on fibronectin-coated plates was inhibited by antibodies to sialyl Lewis[x/a] and E-selectin. E-selectin seems to function in capillary morphogenesis via endothelial cell-cell interaction during angiogenesis. These findings indicate that although ICAM-1 and E-selectin are essential factors, they have a different roles in PMN-induced angiogenesis, i.e., ICAM-1 might act as a signaling receptor for induction of Ets-1 expression, and E-selectin might act in formation of tube-like structure via endothelial cell-cell adhesion.

Recently, it has been known that ICAM-1 plays a role as a signaling receptor though outside-inside signaling events in addition to cell-to-cell adhesion in several different types of cells. To clear the role of ICAM-1 on the PMN-induced angiogenesis, we examined the effects of ICAM-1 cross-linking on angiogenesis using anti-ICAM-1 ligation antibody which mimic adhesion of PMN and endothelial cell. The cross-linking of ICAM-1

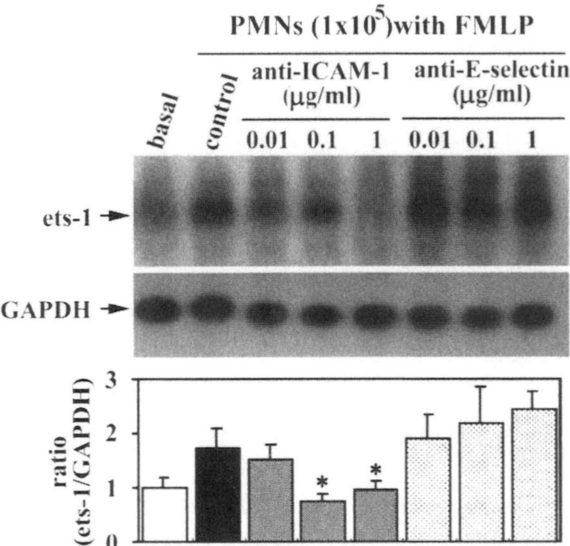

Fig. 3. Effects of antibodies to adhesion molecules on PMN-induced *ets*-1 mRNA expression in BAECs. BAECs were starved of serum for 48 h and pretreated with 0.01–1 µg/mL anti-E-selectin or anti-ICAM-1 antibody. Subsequently, the BAECs were stimulated with 1×10^5 PMNs/mL stimulated with 1 µM FMLP for 3 h before RNA extraction. After electrophoresis of 20 µg RNA/sample and transfer onto nylon membranes, the blots were sequentially hybridized with ^{32}P-labeled *ets*-1 cDNA (*top*) and GAPDH cDNA (*bottom*) probes. Each column indicates the means ± SE ratio of *ets*-1 mRNA expression to GAPDH mRNA from 4 independent experiments. *$P < 0.05$ vs. control.

increased angiogenesis compared with control (Fig. 4a and b). However, the treatment with IgG (Fig. 4c) or ICAM-1 alone (data not shown) did not induce significant changes of the morphology. These result indicated a novel effect of ICAM-1 in the facilitation of angiogenesis.

4 Conclusion

PMN adhesion to ECs induced angiogenesis via ICAM-1, and the induction mechanisms was related with the transcription factor, ets-1 expression mediated by H_2O_2. The direct ICAM-1 stimulation induced by ICAM-1 cross-linking on EC by using anti-ICAM-1 ligation antibody stimulated

90

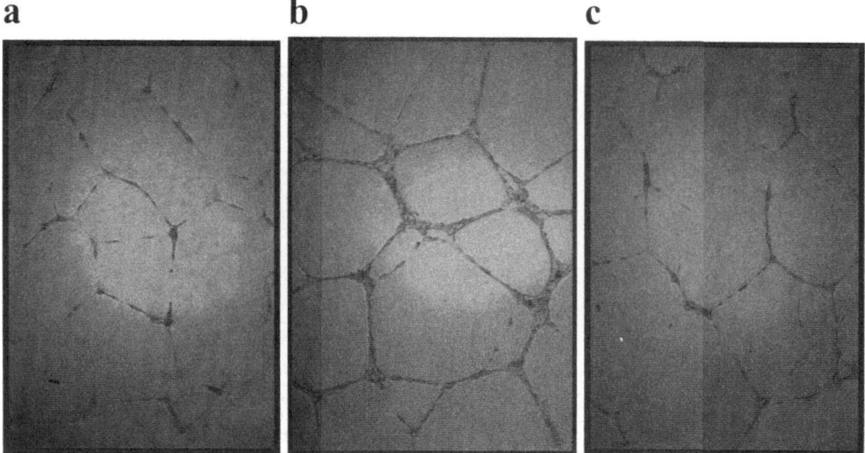

Fig. 4. Typical photographs of angiogenesis after ICAM-1 cross-linking. HUVECs
(5×10^4 cells/mL) were inoculated on Matrigel. The HUVECs were incubated with
(b) or without (a) anti-ICAM-1 antibodies for 30 min. After incubation, the cells
were washed with PBS, and then incubated with or without IgG (10 μg/mL).
HUVECs were treated with or without (control) 1 μg/mL anti-ICAM-1 antibodies,
and then added 10 μg/mL IgG (ICAM-1). "IgG" was added IgG only (c). Magnification is ×40.

angiogenesis, as a result, it was revealed that ICAM-1 plays an important
role on angiogenesis. The results give suggestions that a part of induction mechanisms of angiogenesis is regulated by transcription factor ets-1
expression which induces integrin β_3 (Yasuda et al. 2004) or MMPs
concerned with angiogenesis and the expression is mediated by H_2O_2
(Fig. 5). The potentiation of angiogenesis mediated by ICAM-1 may play an
important role in angiogenesis which is observed in the healing process or
inflammation.

Acknowledgment

We thank Dr. Shinji Naito for cDNA primer of ets-1 and Dr. Yasuna
Kobayashi, Dr. Noriko Kohyama, Dr. Daisuke Kamei, Yumi Ohzeki, Kyoko
Ohhinata, Tomokazu Suzuki, and Mie Ozawa for technical assistance and
discussions.

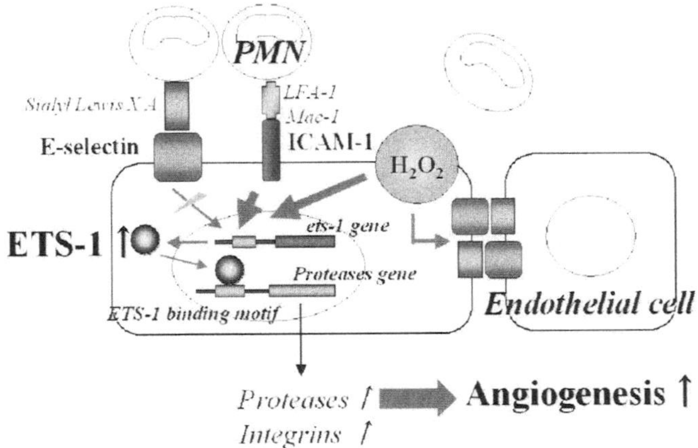

Fig. 5. The diagram summarizes PMN-induced angiogenesis. PMN adhesion to ECs via ICAM-1 might induce angiogenesis by the regulation of integrin or proteases concerned with angiogenesis following transcription factor ets-1 mediated by H_2O_2. The direct stimulation of ICAM-1 by using anti-ICAM-1 antibody stimulated angiogenesis, as a result, it was revealed that ICAM-1 might act as a signaling receptor for induction of Ets-1 expression, and E-selectin might act in formation of tube-like structures via endothelial cell-cell adhesion.

References

Babior BM, Kipnes RS, Curnutte JT (1973) Biological defense mechanisms; The production by leukocytes of superoxide, a potential bactericidal agent. J Clin Invest 52:741–744

Barchowsky A, Munro SR, Morana SJ, Vincenti MP, Treadwell M (1995) Oxidant-sensitive and phosphorylation-dependent activation of NF-kappa B and AP-1 in endothelial cells. Am J Physiol 269:L829–836

Del Maschio A, Zanetti A, Corada M, Rival Y, Ruco L, Lampugnani MG, Dejana E (1996) Polymorphonuclear leukocyte adhesion triggers the disorganization of endothelial cell-to-cell adherens junction. J Cell Biol 135:497–510

Del Zoppo GJ (1997) Microvascular responses to cerebral ischemia/inflammation. Ann NY Acad Sci 823:132–147

Durieu-Trautmann O, Chaverot N, Cazaubon S, Strosberg AD, Couraud PO (1994) Intercellular adhesion molecule 1 activation induces tyrosine phosphorylation of the cytoskeleton-associated protein cortactin in brain microvessel endothelial cells. J Biol Chem 269:12536–12540

Folkman J (1995) Angiogenesis in cancer, vascular, rheumatoid and other disease. Nat Med 1:27–31

Gasic AC, McGuire G, Krater S, Farhood AI, Goldstein MA, Smith CW, Entman M, Taylor AA (1991) Hydrogen peroxide pretreatment of perfused canine vessels induces ICAM-1 and CD18-dependent neutrophil adherence. Circulation 84:2154–2166

Hoffstein ST, Gennaro DE, Manzi RM (1985) Neutrophils may directly synthesize both H_2O_2 and O_2^- since surface stimuli induce their release in stimulus-specific ratios. Inflammation 9: 425–437

Irani K (2000) Oxidant signaling in vascular cell growth, death, and survival: a review of the roles of reactive oxygen species in smooth muscle and endothelial cell mitogenic and apoptotic signaling. Cir Res 87:179–183

Iwasaka C, Tanaka K, Abe M, and Sato Y (1996) Ets-1 regulates angiogenesis by inducing the expression of urokinase-type plasminogen activator and matrix metalloproteinase-1 and the migration of vascular endothelial cells. J Cell Physiol 169:522–531

Jackson JR, Seed MP, Kircher CH, Willoughby DA, Winkler JD (1997) The codependence of angiogenesis and chronic inflammation. FASEB J 11:457–465

Koch AE, Harlow LA, Haines GK, Amento EP, Uemori EN, Wong WL, Pope RM, Ferrara N (1994) Vascular endothelial growth factor. A cytokine modulating endothelial function in rheumatoid arthritis. I Immunol 152:4149–4156

Koch AE, Polverini PJ, Kunkel SL, Harlow LA, Dipietro DA, Elner VM, Elner SG, Strieter RM (1992) Interleukin-8 as a macrophage-derived mediator of angiogenesis. Science 258:1798–1801

Koch AE, Polverini PJ, Leibovich SJ (1986) Induction of neovascularization by activated human monocytes. J Leukoc Biol 39:233–238

Kopprasch S, Gatzweiler A, Kohl M Schroder HE (1995) Endothelin-1 does not prime polymorphonuclear leukocytes for enhanced production of reactive oxygen metabolites. Inflammation 19:679–687

Lo SK, Everitt J, Gu J, Malik AB (1992) Tumor necrosis factor mediates experimental pulmonary edema by ICAM-1 and CD18-dependent mechanisms. J Clin Invest 89:981–988

Lorenzon P, Vecile E, Nardon E, Ferrero E, Harlan JM, Tedesco F, Dobrina A (1998) Endothelial cell E- and P-selectin and vascular cell adhesion molecule-1 function as signaling receptors. J Cell Biol 142:1381–1391

Nguyen M, Strubel NA, Bischoff J (1993) A role for sialyl Lewis-X/A glycoconjugates in capillary morphogenesis. Nature 365:267–269

Oda N, Abe M, Sato Y (1999) ETS-1 converts endothelial cells to the angiogenic phenotype by inducing the expression of matrix metalloproteinases and integrin beta3. J Cell Physiol 178:121–132

Sato Y (1998) Transcription factor ETS-1 as a molecular target for angiogenesis inhibition. Hum Cell 11:207–214

Sunderkotter C, Steinbrink K, Goebeler M, Bhardwaj R, Sorg C (1994) Macrophage and angiogenesis. J Leukoc Biol 55:410–422

Vissers MC, Day WA, Winterbourn CC (1985) Neutrophils adherent to a nonphagocytosable surface (glomerular basement membrane) produce oxidants only at the site of attachment. Blood 66:161–166

Wang Q, Doesrschuk CM (2002) The signaling pathway induced by neutrophil-endothelial cell adhesion. Antioxid Redox Signal 4:39–47

Weissmann G, Smolen JE, Korchak HM (1980) Release of inflammatory mediators from stimulated neutrophils. N Engl J Med 303:27–349

Yasuda M, Shimizu S, Tokuyama S, Watanabe T, Kiuchi Y YamamotoT (2000) A novel effect of polymorphonuclear leukocytes in the facilitation of angiogenesis. Life Sci 66:2113–2121

Yasuda M, Ohbayashi M, Ohhinata K, Yamamoto T (2004) The involvement of integrin $\alpha v \beta_3$ in polymorphonuclear leukocyte-induced angiogenesis in bovine aortic endothelial cells. Life Sci 75:421–434

Yasuda M, Ohzeki Y, Shimizu S, Naito S, Ohtsuru A, Yamamoto T, Kuroiwa Y (1999) Stimulation of in vitro angiogenesis by hydrogen peroxide and the relation with ets-1 in endothelial cells. Life Sci 64:249–258

Yasuda M, Shimizu S, Ohhinata K, Naito S, Tokuyama S, Mori Y, Kiuchi Y, Yamamoto T (2002) Differential roles of ICAM-1 and E-selectin in polymorphonuclear leukocyte-induced angiogenesis. Am J Physiol Cell Physiol 282:C917–C925

Improvement of severe ulcer of buerger's disease by bone-marrow mononuclear cell transplantation: a case report

Teruko Soda[1], Hiroshi Suzuki[1]*, Taro Kusuyama[1], Yuya Yokota[1],
Yasutoshi Omori[1], Takatoshi Sato[1], Fumiyoshi Tsunoda[1], Makoto Shoji[1],
Yoshitaka Iso[1], Shinji Koba[1], Eiichi Geshi[1], Takashi Katagiri[1],
Shigeru Tomoyasu[2]

[1]Third Department of Internal Medicine and [2]Department of Hematology,
Showa University School of Medicine, 1-5-8 Hatanodai, Shinagawa-ku,
Tokyo 142-8555, Japan

Summary. [Case Report]A 47-year-old man with Buerger's disease was admitted with complaints of progressive ulcer of left planta pedis and resting pain of the left leg. The ulcer was not healed under medical therapy nor lumbar sympathetic ganglion block, and angioplasty or bypass surgery was not applicable. All his toes showed cyanotic and left third and fifth toes were gangrene, as well as ulcer in left planta pedis. Angiography showed arterial occlusion in the crus and formation of corkscrew like changes. Although ankle-brachial index was kept in almost normal range, transcutaneous oxygen pressure (TcO_2) was decreased. Leg pain was not relieved with medication and he could not walk for pain due to his ulcer. We performed bone-marrow mononuclear cell implantation to his inferior limbs to achieve therapeutic angiogenesis. After aspirating the bone marrow (600 ml) from the ileum, the bone-marrow mononuclear cells were sorted. The separated cells were implanted into the ischemic legs by intramuscular injection. Reduction of leg pain was observed as early as 3 days, and completely disappeared at rest after 4 weeks. Improvement of TcO_2 was observed at 1 week, and the ulcer of planta pedis was almost healed 4 weeks after the therapy. [Conclusion] Bone-marrow mononuclear cell implantation is very effective in patients with Buerger's disease, even they have large severe ulcer.

Key words. bone-marrow mononuclear cell, cell implantation, transcutaneous oxygen pressure, peripheral artery disease

1 Introduction

Autologous bone marrow mononuclear cell (BM-MNC) implantaion into ischemic limbs has recently been developed as a therapeutic angiogenesis for patients with severe peripheral artery disease who are not be good candidates of percutaneous transluminal angioplasty or bypass surgery (Tateishi-Yuyama and Matsubara et al. 2002, Higashi and Kimura et al. 2004, Saigawa and Kato et al. 2004). The results so far reported on this new therapeutic approach have been promising (Tateishi-Yuyama and Matsubara et al. 2002, Higashi and Kimura et al. 2004, Saigawa and Kato et al. 2004), but number of patients treated with this therapy is still small. In theory, the commitment of CD34-positive endothelial progenitor cells to vessel formation, so-called vasculogenesis, is thought to be the main mechanism behind the angiogenic effect (Asahara and Murohara et al. 1997).

We report a case of Burger's disease with large and intractable leg ulcer whose symptom was cured early after BM-MNC implantaion.

2 Case report

A 47-year-old man whose chief complaint was progressive ischemic change, ulcer of left planta pedis and resting pain of the left leg was admitted to our hospital to receive bone marrow cell implantation. From 1997, his bilateral inferior limb ache and a ulcer of left planta pedis were developed, and he was diagnosed as Buerger's disease by angiography. The ulcer was not healed in medical treatment or lumbar sympathetic ganglion block, and was not suitable for angioplasty or bypass surgery. As past history, he had gall bladder resection at the age of 42, and suffered from duodenal ulcer perforation at the age of 46. He had smoked 30 cigarettes per day until 45 years old. Even after he was diagnosed as Buerger's disease, he has still been smoking seven or eight cigarettes per day. On risk factor for peripheral artery disease, he suffered from hypercholesterolemia, taking 3-hydroxy-3-methlglutaryl coenzyme A reductase inhibitor every day. Each his toe and heel was cyanotic, and left third and fifth toes were gangrene, as well as ulcer in left planta pedis (30 mm × 15 mm). Rest pain scale of his leg was 3. Rest pain scale was determined in Trial for Therapeutic Angiogenesis Using Cell Transplantation (Tateishi-Yuyama and Matsubara et al. 2002) as following. The scale is evaluated by subjective symptom. +4: severe pain unresolved with paracetamol or NSAID (non-steroid anti-inflammatory drug), +3: moderate pain NSAID necessary, +2: slight pain NSAID unnecessary, +1: very slight pain, 0: completely resolved. Angiography showed occlusion of crus trifurcation and corkscrew like formation below the occlusion site in his both legs His right ankle-brachial index (ABI) was 0.89, and left one was 0.86. His peripheral transcutaneous oxygen pressure (TcO_2) was decreased in dorsalis pedis; crus; 51 mmHg (rt.), 55 mmHg (lt.), dorsalis pedis; 21 mmHg (rt.), and 27 mmHg (lt.). As for treadmil test (Inclination zero degree, 3 km/h), he couldn't walk at all.

The procedure of BM-MNC implantation was almost the same as that previously described (Tateishi-Yuyama and Matsubara et al. 2002). After aspirating the bone marrow (600 ml) from the ileum under general anesthesia, the BM-MNCs were sorted on a CS3000-Plus blood-cell separator (Baxter International Inc., Deerfield, IL, USA), and concentrated to a final volume of 60 ml. The separated cells were implanted into the ischemic areas of both legs by intramuscular injection using 26 G needles.

A number of BM-MNC was calculated by manually counting and CD34-positive cells were counted using a fluorescence-activated cell sorter. The drugs used were not changed throughout the hospitalization.

The number of injected cells was 3.48×10^9. The mean number of CD34-positive cells was 3.35×10^7 (0.8% of the injected cells).

Angiographc findings and ABI were not improved, however, TcO_2 improved as early as 1 week and increased to 50 mmHg at 4 weeks, further improving to 57 mmHg at 1 year after the BM-MNC implantation (Fig. 1). Rest pain scale also improved from as early as 3 days, and he remained free

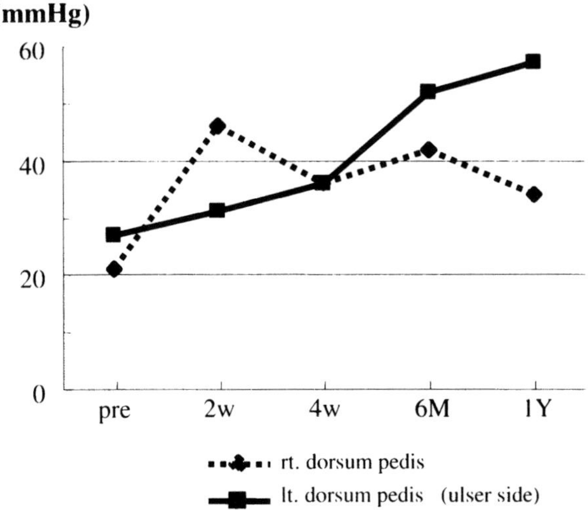

Fig. 1. Changes in transcutaneous oxygen pressure (TcO2) between baseline and 4 weeks after bone-marrow mononuclear cell implantation. TcO2; transcutaneous oxygen pressure.

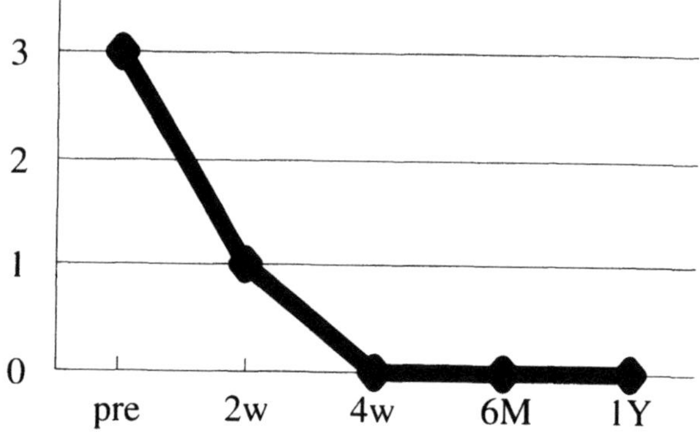

Fig. 2. Rest pain scale. Rest pain scale was improved significantly from early stage.

from leg pain at 1 year (Fig. 2). Although he couldn't walk at all in Treadmil's test before the BM-MNC implantation because of leg pain, he was able to walk as long as 45 minutes after the therapy. Severe and intractable ulcer of planta pedis was almost healed at 4 weeks and was completely cured after 6 months of the therapy (Fig. 3), keeping the therapeutic effects more than 1 year.

3 Discussion

We experienced a case of Burger's disease with large and intractable leg ulcer whose symptom was cured early after BM-MNC implantation.

In theory, the commitment of CD34-positive endothelial progenitor cells to vessel formation, so-called vasculogenesis, is thought to be the main mechanism behind the angiogenic effect (Asahara and Murohara et al. 1997). However, CD34-positive cells make up only a very small population among the BM-MNCs. As it turns out, sorted BM-MNC fraction contains not only CD34-positive cells, but also an abundance of CD34-negative cells, which release a large amount of cytokines including vascular endothelial growth factor and basic fibroblast growth factor (Tateishi-Yuyama and Matsubara et al. 2002). In this reported case, the size of the large ulcer reduced as early as 1 week, and remarkably decreased at 4 weeks after the therapy. Vasculogenesis induced by endothelial progenitor cells included in CD34-positive cells is considered to require some time to create new microvessels. Early improvement of the ulcer and other symptoms suggest the great contribution of pro-angiogenic cytokines such as vascular endothelial growth factor, basic fibroblast growth factor, hepatocyte growth factor and interleukin 1β included mainly CD34-negative cells in the BM-MNC implantation as a new mechanism.

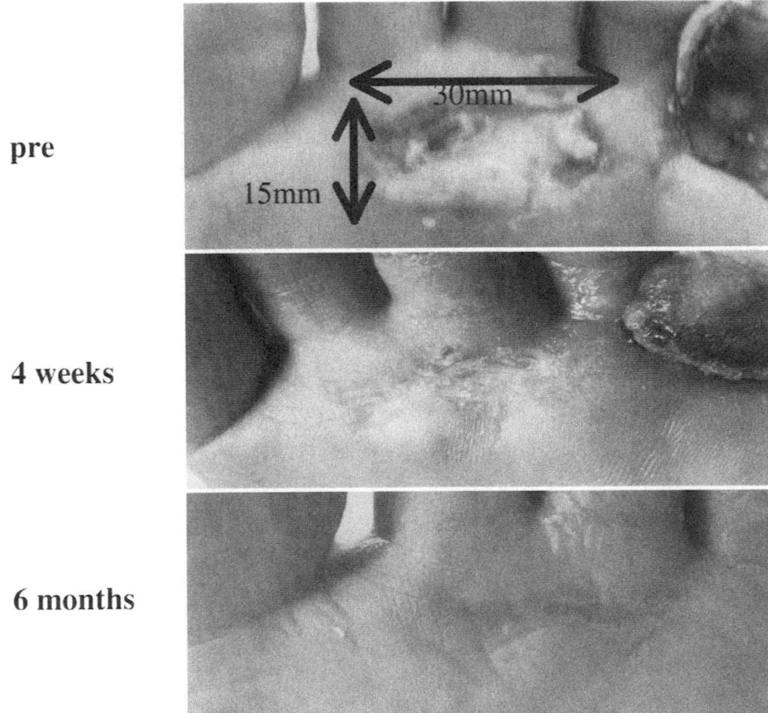

Fig. 3. Ulcer healing process. Macroscopic findings; intractable ulcer sized 30 mm × 15 mm healed within 4 weeks. And after 6 months, ulcer scar also disappeared.

4 Conclusion

BM-MNC implantation is very effective in patients with Buerger's disease, even they have large severe ulcer.

References

Asahara T, Murohara T, Sullivan A, Silver M, van der Zee R, Li T, et al. (1997) Isolation of putative progenitor endothelial cells for angiogenesis. Science 275:964–7

Higashi Y, Kimura M, Hara K, Noma K, Jitsuiki D, Nakagawa K, et al. (2004) Autologous bone-marrow mononuclear cell implantation improves endothelium-dependent vasodilation in patients with limb ischemia. Circulation 109:1215–8

Masaki H, et al. (2002) Therapeutic angiogenesis for patients with limb ischaemia by autologous transplantation of bone-marrow cells: a pilot study and a randomized controlled trial. Lancet 360:427–35

Saigawa T, Kato K, Ozawa T, Toba K, Makiyama Y, Minagawa S, et al. (2004) Clinical application of bone marrow implantation in patients with arteiosclerosis obliterans, and the association between efficacy and the number of implanted bone marrow cells. Circ J 68:1189–93

Scheffler A, Rieger H. (1992) A comparative analysis of transcutanoeous oximetry (tcPO$_2$) during oxygen inhalation and leg dependency in severe peripheral arterial occlusive disease. J Vasc Surg. 16:18–24

Cardioprotective effect of G-CSF administration after coronary reperfusion in swine AMI model

Takatoshi Sato[1], Hiroshi Suzuki[1], Taro Kusuyama[1], Yasutoshi Omori[1], Teruko Soda[1], Fumiyoshi Tsunoda[1], Makoto Shoji[1], Yoshitaka Iso[1], Shinji Koba[1], Eiichi Geshi[1], Takashi Katagiri[1], Keisuke Kawachi[2], Kohei Wakabayashi[2], Youich Takeyama[2]

[1]Third Department of Internal Medicine, Showa University School of Medicine, 1-5-8 Hatanodai, Shinagawa-ku, Tokyo 142-8555, Japan
[2]Division of Cardiology, Department of Internal Medicine, Showa University Fujigaoka Hospital, 1-30 Fujigaoka, Aoba-ku, Yokohama, Kanagawa 227-8501, Japan

Summary. [Purpose] Recent studies have suggested that granulocyte colony-stimulating factor (G-CSF) may accelerate angiogenesis or cardio-myogenesis. No previous studies, however, have used large animal models to investigete how clinical doses of G-CSF affect cardiac function after acute myocardial infarction (AMI). [Methods] Diagonal branch of the left anterior descending coronary artery of domestic swine was balloon-occluded for 1-hour and then reperfused. The G-CSF group received a subcutaneous injection of G-CSF at a dose of $5.0\,\mu g/kg/day$ for 6 days after MI. Left ventriculography was performed 4 weeks after MI. The number of vessels in the infarcted area were calculated using sections stained by anti-α-smooth muscle actin (SMA) and anti-von Willebrand factor (vWF). Reverse transcription polymerase chain reactions for collagen I, collagen III, and transforming growth factor (TGF)-β were also examined. [Results] The G-CSF group showed a significantly higher ejection fraction and lower end-diastolic volume in left ventriculography. The numbers of α-SMA- and vWF-positive vessels in the G-CSF group were significantly larger. The expression of collagen III mRNA was significantly lower in the G-CSF group in the infarct and border areas. The expression of TGF-β mRNA was significantly lower in the G-CSF group in the border area. [Conclusions] The administration of clinical doses of G-CSF improved cardiac function after reperfusion in AMI. G-CSF confers its effects by accelerating angio-genesis and modifying the wound-healing process.

102

Key words. Angiogenesis, transforming growth factor-β, collagen I, collagen III

The mobilization of bone marrow stem cells by cytokines may be a promising strategy for repairing the infarcted myocardium. Granulocyte colony-stimulating factor (G-CSF) and several other growth factors have been reported to mobilize hematopoietic precursor cells from the bone marrow (1, 2, 3) and to stimulate endothelial cell migration and proliferation (4). G-CSF is one of the most thoroughly studied growth factors in the setting of MI. G-CSF stimulates the proliferation and differentiation of precursor cells committed to the neutrophil/granulocyte cell type (5). Several studies on G-CSF treatment after MI have demonstrated improvements in cardiac function, reductions of left ventricular (LV) remodeling, and improvements in LV function (6, 7, 8, 9, 10). Other recent results, however, have dampened the enthusiasm about G-CSF and shed doubt on the capacity of growth factors to induce regeneration and neovascularization of myocardial tissue (10, 11,12). As of this writing, only two earlier reports have focused on the effects of G-CSF in large animals, one in a permanent occlusion model (13) and the other in a chronic myocardial ischemia model (14). In this study we investigated how G-CSF administration influenced cardiac function after AMI in a swine model of ischemia reperfusion.

1 Methods

1.1 Animal experimental protocol

The current study was performed according to the Guide for the Care and Use of Laboratory Animals published by the US National Institute of Health. The experimental protocol was approved by the Animal Care and Use Committee of the Showa University School of Medicine. The experiments were performed using 17 male domestic pigs. The procedure was performed by inserting an introducer from the right cervical artery, feeding balloon catheter through the introducer into the first diagonal branch of the left anterior descending coronary artery, inflating the catheter for 60 minutes to induce MI, and reperfusing the vessel. Each animal in the G-CSF group (n = 9) received a subcutaneous injection of G-CSF at a dose of 5.0 μg/kg daily for 6 days, starting from just after reperfusion, and each control animal (n = 8) received same volume of saline. Left ventriculography was performed before and 4 weeks after MI to determine cardiac function. Later, upon the completion of follow-up coronary angiography and left ventriculography at 4 weeks after MI, the animals were sacrificed and their hearts were harvested.

1.2 Tissue preparation and immunohistochemistry

The animals were sacrificed at 4 weeks after MI, and their hearts were excised. Samples were collected from each of three areas in each excised heart (infarcted area, risk area, and remote area). Some of the samples were frozen in liquid nitrogen for extraction of mRNA. Others were fixed in a 10% formalin solution for 24 h and embedded in paraffin for morphometric analysis. Sequential 4- to 5-μm-thick traverse sections were cut, affixed to glass slides, stained with hematoxylin, eosin, and Mallory staining for immunohistochemistry.

The sections were deparaffinized and subjected to a 3-step immunostaining procedure using a streptavidin-biotin complex with horseradish peroxidase. Horseradish peroxidase activity was visualized with a diaminobenzidine substrate and the sections were faintly counterstained with hematoxylin. The primary antibodies were anti-α-smooth muscle actin (SMA) for small arteries and anti-von Willebrand factor (vWF) for endothelial cells. The numbers of α-SMA- and vWF- positive vessels in the infarcted areas were manually counted in each section for immunohistochemistry.

1.3 Tissue preparation for transcription-polymerase chain reaction for collagen I, collagen III, and TGF-ß

Reverse transcription-polymerase chain reaction (RT-PCR) analyses were performed for collagen I, collagen III, and TGF-ß. Total RNA was extracted from frozen samples by the modified acid guanidinium thiocyanate/phenol/chloroform method. The RNA concentration and purity were estimated spectrophotometrically and the quality was further assessed using an Agilent 2100 Bioanalyzer (Agilent Technologies, Palo Alto, CA, USA).

Total RNA was subjected to RT-PCR analysis. cDNA was synthesized from RNA by the following method. Total RNA (1 μg), random hexamer (Applied Biosystems, Foster City, CA, USA), and the manufacturer's recommended buffer were mixed and incubated at 95°C for 2 min, cooled to 37°C, and incubated with Superscript II (Invitrogen, Carlsbad, CA, USA), 10 mmol/L dithiothreitol, 0.5 mmol/L of each dNTP, and 20U RNAs (Promega, Madison, WI, USA) at 42°C for 50 min. Previously described methods were used to prepare the primer sequences for PCR and to perform the PCR itself (15). The sizes and quantities of the PCR products were detected by Agilent 2100 Bioanalyzer (Agilent Technologies).

104

1.4 Statistical analysis

All values are expressed as means ± SEM. The means were compared by the unpaired Student's t-test. A P value of less than 0.05 was considered statistically significant.

2 Results

2.1 Left ventriculography

The G-CSF group had a significantly higher ejection fraction (43.5 ± 4.7% (control) vs. 49.1 ± 5.9% (G-CSF), P < 0.05; Figure 1A) and significantly lower left ventricular end-diastolic volume (37.9 ± 7.5 ml (control) vs. 27.9 ± 8.7 ml (G-CSF), P < 0.05; Figure 1B) in comparison with the control at the 4-week ventriculography.

2.2 Immunohistochemical analysis

VWF- and α-SMA-positive vessels were counted in the infarcted areas. The G-CSF group had significantly greater numbers of vWF-positive vessels (283.5 ± 455.5/mm^2 (control) vs. 555.9 ± 326.1/mm^2 (G-CSF), P < 0.005; Figures 2A) and α-SMA-positive vessels (7.4 ± 2.5/mm^2 (control) vs. 16.3 ± 7.8/mm^2 (G-CSF), P < 0.05; Figures 2B).

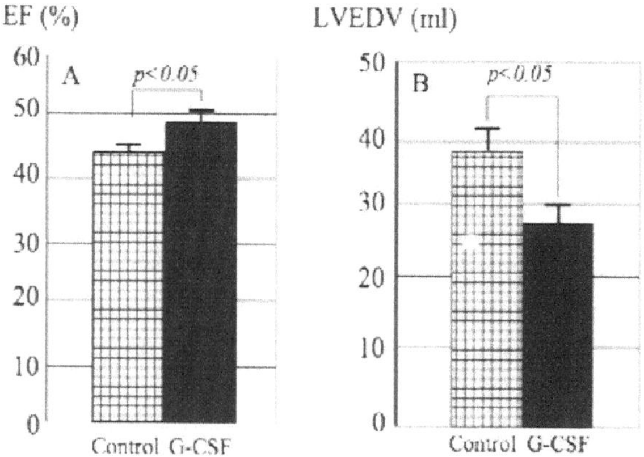

Fig. 1. Left ventriculography data at 4 weeks after MI. EF indicates ejection fraction (A); LVEDV, left ventricular end-diastolic volume (B).

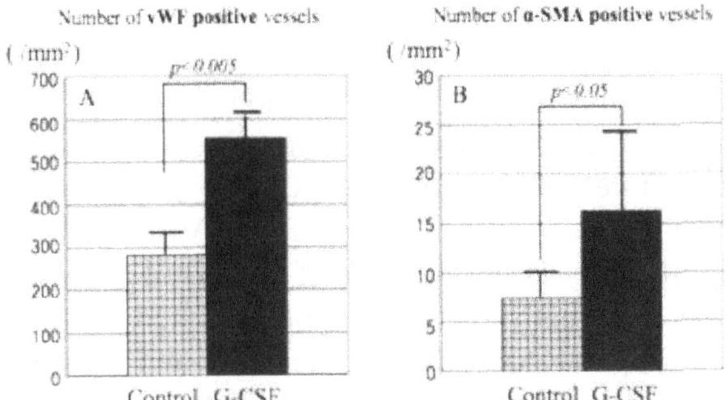

Fig. 2. Vessel density. A; number of vWF-positive vessels. B; number of α-SMA-positive vessels.

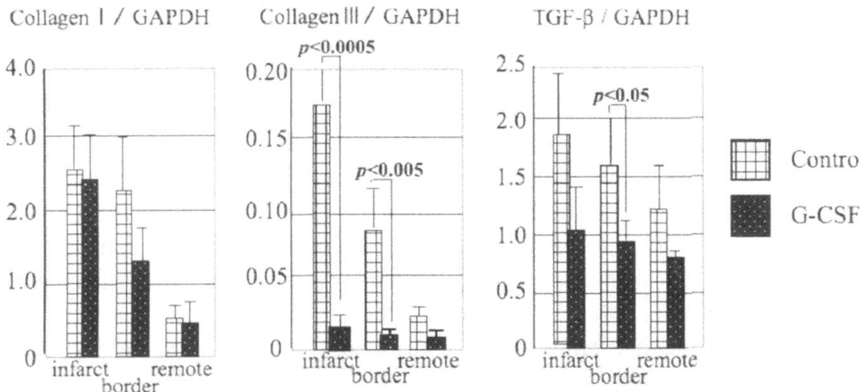

Fig. 3. RT-PCR for collagen I, collagen III, TGF-β.

2.3 PCR analysis

The expressions of collagen I, collagen III, and TGF-β mRNA were evaluated by the PCR method in the infarct, border, and remote areas (Figure 3). The expression of collagen I mRNA in the border area tended to be weaker in the G-CSF group than in the control, but the difference was not significant. The expression of collagen III mRNA in the G-CSF group was significantly weaker in both the infarct ($P < 0.0005$) and border ($P < 0.005$) areas. In the border area it tended to be weaker, but the difference was not significant. TGF-β mRNA expression in the infarct and remote areas did not significantly differ between the groups, but it tended to be smaller in the G-CSF group. In the border area it was significantly weaker in the G-CSF group ($P < 0.05$).

3 Discussion

The findings of the present study demonstrated the effectiveness of G-CSF in improving cardiac function in a swine MI model after coronary reperfusion. In left ventriculography, the G-CSF group exhibited a significantly higher EF and a significantly smaller LVEDV. The G-CSF group exhibited a significantly larger number of vessels in the vWF and α-SMA stainings. In the PCR analysis, the control exhibited significantly stronger expression of TGF-β mRNA in the border area and significantly stronger expression of collagen III mRNA in the infarct and border areas, compared to G-CSF group.

Several studies have confirmed the effectiveness of G-CSF in improving cardiac function, preventing LV remodeling, and improving LV function after MI (6, 7, 8, 9, 13, 16). Treatment with G-CSF reduced LV remodeling and improved cardiac function in mouse (6) and swine (13) models of permanent occlusion after MI. G-CSF-treated animals exhibited a smaller LV dimension, increased LV ejection fraction, and thicker infarct-LV wall than control animals in a rabbit coronary occlusion and reperfusion model of MI (7). None of these earlier studies were immediately similar to the actual clinical setting, however, as they were performed using either small animal models or a large animal model of permanent occlusion. The present study is the first to demonstrate the effect of G-CSF in preventing LV remodeling and improving LV function using a large animal model after coronary reperfusion of MI.

One possible mechanism behind the improvements in LV remodeling and LV function conferred by G-CSF after MI may be the angiogenic effect. Our vWF and α-SMA stainings showed more vessels in the G-CSF group than in the control group. This meant that the G-CSF treatment induced angiogenesis at the small arterial levels as well as the microcapillary level. Likewise, several other groups have reported G-CSF induced angiogenesis in experimental models of MI (3, 6, 13, 16). G-CSF has been found to mobilize hematopoietic precursor cells from the bone marrow (1, 2, 3) and to stimulate endothelial cell migration and proliferation (4). In fact, the mobilization of bone marrow stem cells to the myocardium has been described as the main mechanism behind the G-CSF-induced angiogenesis (17, 18). The direct effects of G-CSF in reducing the apoptotic cell death of cardiomyocytes and endothelial cells may be another mechanism behind the improvement in cardiac function and induction of angiogenesis (6, 16).

Modulation of left ventricular remodeling through the prevention of fibrosis on healing process occurred after MI is also likely to have an important bearing on G-CSF administration. According to our PCR results, the mRNA expressions of collagen III and TGF-β were weaker in the G-CSF-treated animals than in the control at 4 weeks. The weaker expressions of these proteins possibly led to the decreased fibrotic area and the wall thinning, resulting in the inhibition of the left ventricular expansion reflected by the decrease in the left ventricular end-diastolic volume. Two studies demonstrated enhancements in the levels of mRNA expression of TGF-ß, collagen I, and collagen III mRNAs in the infarcted heart after MI, and these enhancements were accelerated by G-CSF administration in the acute stage (8, 9). In both studies, however, the differences in mRNA expression were only significant in the early stage after MI. In the study by Sugano et al. (9), the mRNA expressions of TGF-ß, procollagen I, and procollagen III were similar in the control and G-CSF-treated groups on day 14. The mRNA expressions of those proteins were only measured at 4 weeks after MI in the present study. If we had obtained the data in the earlier stage, we might have observed enhanced expressions in G-CSF-treated group. Minatoguchi et al. (7) reported results similar to our own using a rabbit model of AMI. Specifically, their G-CSF-treated animals exhibited a decreased fibrotic area compared to the controls at 14 days and at 3 months after MI. Decreased protein expressions of proMMP-1 and 9 in their G-CSF-treated group might have led to the post-MI inhibition of fibrosis (7). G-CSF improved cardiac function and inhibited left ventricular remodeling after MI by modifying the wound-healing process and reducing the fibrotic area.

4 Conclusion

The administration of clinical doses of G-CSF after reperfusion in AMI improved cardiac function and prevented left ventricular remodeling in the chronic stage. We propose that G-CSF confers its effects by accelerating angiogenesis and modifying the wound-healing process.

References

1. Laterveer L, Lindley IJ, Hamilton MS, Willemze R, Fibbe WE. Interleukin-8 induces rapid mobilization of hematopoietic stem cells with radioprotective capacity and long term myelolymphoid repopulating ability. Blood 1995;85: 2269–75
2. Lapidot T, Petit I. Current understanding of stem cell mobilization the roles of chemokines, proteolytic enzymes, adhesion molecules, cytokines, and stromal cells. Exp Hematol 2002;30:973–81
3. Orlic D, Kajstura J, Chimenti S, Limana F, Jakoniuk I, Quaini F et al. Mobilized bone marrow cells repair the infarcted heart, improving function and survival. Proc Natl Acad Sci USA 2001;98:10344–9

4. Bussolino F, Wang JM, Defilippi P, Turrini F, Sanavio F, Edgell CJ, et al. Granulocyte- and granulocyte-macrophage-colony stimulating factors induce human endothelial cells to migrate and proliferate. Nature 1989;337:471–3

5. Welte K, Bonilla MA, Gillio AP, Bonne TC, Potter GK, Gabrilove JL, et al. Recombinant human granulocyte colony-stimulating factor effects on hematopoiesis in normal and cyclophosphamide-treated primates. J Exp Med 1987; 165:941–8

6. Ohtuska M, Takano H, Zou Y, Toko H, Akazawa H, Qin Y, et al. Cytokine therapy prevents left ventricular remodeling and dysfunction after myocardial infarction through neovascularization. FASEB J 2004;18:851–3

7. Minatoguchi S, Takemura G, Chen XH, Wang N, Uno Y, Koda M, et al. Acceleration of the healing process and myocardial regeneration may be important as a mechanism of improvement of cardiac function and remodeling by postinfarction granulocyte colony-stimulating factor treatment. Circulation 2004;109: 2572–80

8. Miki T, Miura T, Nishino Y, Yano T, Sakamoto J, Nakamura Y, et al. Granulocyte colony stimulating factor/macrophage colony stimulationg factor improves postinfarct ventricular function by suppression of border zone remodeling in rats. Clin Exp Pharmaco Physiol 2004;31:873–82

9. Sugano Y, Anzai T, Yoshikawa T, Maekawa Y, Kohno T, Mahara K, et al. Granulocyte colony-stimulating factor attenuates early ventricular expansion after experimental myocardial infarction. Cardiovasc Res 2005;65:446–56

10. Maekawa Y, Anzai T, Yoshikawa T, Sugano Y, Mahara K, Kohno T, et al. Effect of granulocyte-macrophage colony-stimulating factor inducer on left ventricular remodeling after acute myocardial infarction. J Am Coll Cardiol 2004;44:1510–20

11. Hill JM, Syed MA, Arai AE, Powell TM, Paul JD, Zalos G, et al. Outcomes and risks of granulocyte colony-stimulating factor in patients with coronary artery disease. J Am Coll Cardiol 2005;46:1643–8

12. Kang HJ, Kim HS, Zhang SY, Park KW, Cho HJ, Koo BK, et al. Effects of intracoronary infusion of peripheral blood stem-cells mobilized with granulocyte-colony stimulating factor on left ventricular systolic function and restenosis after coronary stenting in myocardial infarction: the MAGIC cell randomized clinical trial. Lancet 2004;363:751–6

13. Iwanaga K, Takano H, Ohtsuka M, Hasegawa H, Zou Y, Qin Y, et al. Effect of G-CSF on cardiac remodeling after acute myocardial infarction in swine. Biochem Biophys Res Commun 2004;325:1353–9

14. Hasegawa H, Takano H, Iwanaga K, Ohtsuka M, Qin Y, Niitsuma Y, et al. Cardioprotective effects of granulocyte colony-stimulating factor in swine with chronic myocardial ischemia. J Am Coll Cardiol 2006;47:842–9

15. Wang JF, Olson ME, Reno CR, Kulyk W, Wright JB, Hart DA. Molecular and cell biology of skin wound healing in a pig model. Connect Tissue Res 2000;41:195–211

16. Harada M, Qin Y, Takano H, Minamino T, Zou Y, Toko H, et al. G-CSF prevents cardiac remodeling after myocardial infarction by activating the Jak-Stat pathway in cardiomyocytes. Nature Med 2005;11:305–11

17. Kocher AA, Schuster MD, Szabolcs MJ, Takuma S, Birkhoff D, Wang J, et al. Neovascularization of ischemic myocardium by human bone marrow-derived angioblasts prevents cardiomyocyte apoptosis, reduces remodeling and improves cardiac function. Nature Med 2001;7:430–6
18. Pfeffer MA, Branwald E. Ventricular remodeling after myocardial infarction: experimental observations and clinical implications. Circulation 1990; 81:1161–72

Part III
The Nervous System

Adult neurogenesis in the hippocampus

Tatsunori Seki

Department of Anatomy II, Juntendo University School of Medicine, 2-1-1 Hongo, Bunkyo-ku, Tokyo 113-8421, Japan

Summary. Neurogenesis usually ceases by the early postnatal period. However, exceptional adult neurogenesis occurs in the hippocampus of mammals, including humans. We have been investigating how newly generated neurons develop and add new neuronal circuits to the adult hippocampus. Recently we have focused on the early developmental events of adult neurogenesis and have found the systemic cellular arrangement and intercellular relationship of proliferating neural precursors and migrating neuroblasts.

Key words. Hippocampus, adult neurogenesis, clustering, migration

1 History

For more than 100 years, it was believed that neurons are never generated in the adult brain (Gould and Gross 2002). This paradigm changed in the late 90's and most neuroscientists now believe that neurons continue to be generated in two restricted adult brain regions: the hippocampus and the subventricular zone of the forebrain. However, the phenomenon of adult neurogenesis itself had been discovered in the early 1960's by Altman who used ^{3}H-thymidine autoradiography and labeled nuclei of proliferating cells in the adult rat hippocampus (Altman and Das 1965).

Thereafter, studies on adult neurogenesis by a few scientist groups continued until the early 90's using ^{3}H-thymidine autoradiography. In the late 70's and early 80's, Kaplan revealed with a combination of autoradiography and electron microscopy that the newly generated cells labeled with ^{3}H-thymidine form synapses (Kaplan and Hinds 1977; Kaplan 2001).

In the 80's, Nottenbohn's group studied neurogenesis in adult song birds and found that adult neurogenesis was associated with learning of the bird song (Goldman and Nottbohm 1983). In the early 90's, McEwen's group began to study the influence of stress on adult neurogenesis of the rat hippocampus (Gould et al. 1992).

One of the problems of these ^{3}H-thymidine-autoradiographical studies is that only nuclei are labeled in proliferating cells that incorporate ^{3}H-thymidine during a short period of time after the ^{3}H-thymidine injection. The investigators could not detect the dendrites and axons of newly generated cells at the light microscopic level and also did not know how many developing cells are present in the adult hippocampus. Additionally, autoradiography is time-consuming as it requires a few weeks or up to more than one month to detect ^{3}H-thymidine-labeled cells.

In the early 90's we found that newly generated and developing neurons in the adult hippocampus specifically express polysialic acid (PSA), a carbohydrate portion of neural cell adhesion molecules (NCAM) (Seki and Arai 1991; Seki and Arai 1993). The immunohistochemistry for PSA can visualize the detailed morphology of the dendrites and axons of developing neurons. Additional progress is labeling by bromodeoxyuridine (BrdU), a thymidine analog which was first used in embryonic and postnatal hippocampus by Nowakowski's group (Miller and Nowakowski 1988). We performed double immunohistochemistry for PSA and BrdU in the adult hippocampus, to follow-up the fate of newly generated cells and observe the detailed morphology of the developing neurons (Seki and Arai 1993; Seki and Arai 1995), and thereafter the same method was used by the other group (Kuhn et al. 1996).

Double or triple immunohistochemistry for BrdU and various neural markers became the standard method to study adult neurogenesis in the late 90's. Recently, doublecortin and collapsing response-mediated protein 4 (CRMP-4) have been used as molecular markers for immature neurons in immunohistochemistry. Distributions of doublecortin- and CRMP-4-expressing cells are reported to be similar to that of PSA-expressing cells (Nacher et al. 2001; Seki 2002a). Additionally, a retrovirus vector bearing the green fluorescence protein (GFP) gene is now used to label newly generated cells. Retrovirus vector-GFP labeling allows us to perform living imaging and electrophysiology in slices of brain tissue.

2 Cell proliferation and clustering

The hippocampal formation consists of two neuronal layers: the granule cell layer and pyramidal cell layer. The area of neurogenesis in the adult hippocampal formation is confined to the deepest part of the granule cell layer. Although adult neurogenesis continues in aged rats, the rate of the production of new neurons decreases with aging (Seki and Arai 1995; Kuhn et al. 1996). This suggests that the neurogenic region of the adult hippocampus does not contain real stem cells, but progenitor cells that have limited proliferative property. Actually, *in vitro* neurosphere experiments indicate that the adult hippocampus contains progenitors with limited self-renewal (Seaberg and van Der Kooy 2002).

Progenitor cells of the adult neurogenic regions have been reported to possess astrocytic features and express GFAP in the dentate gyrus (Seri et al. 2001) and the SVZ of the forebrain (Doetsch et al. 1999). Developmental processes of the astrocytic progenitor cells have been proposed (Kempermann et al. 2004). The first GFAP-expressing neural progenitors are considered to divide slowly and to extend radial processes. The second neuronal precursors that express some neuronal markers, such as PSA and doublecortin, proliferate quickly and the majority are tangentially oriented cells. The first neural progenitors and the second neuronal precursors have different electrophysiological properties (Filippov et al. 2003; Fukuda et al. 2003). However, the exact morphology and cellular arrangement of these neural progenitor and precursor cells remain to be explored.

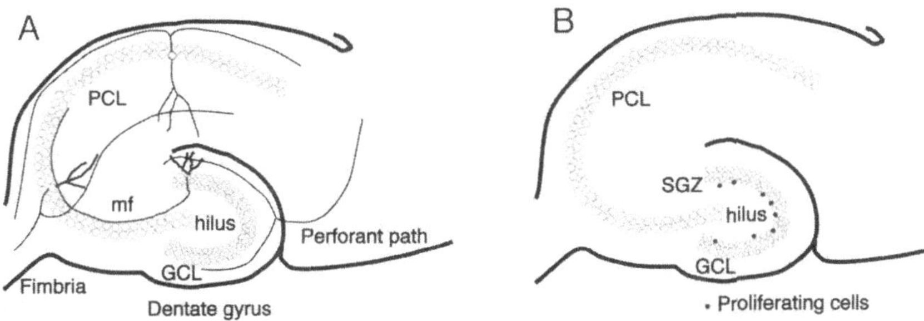

Fig. 1. Neuronal circuits (A) and neurogenic region (B) of the adult hippocampus. Neurons continue to be generated in the innermost part of the granule cell layer (GCL) or subgranular zone (SGZ). mf, mossy fibers; PCL, pyramidal cell layer.

We have examined the cellular arrangements of the newly generated cells using BrdU labeling and PSA immunohistochemistry. In the dentate neurogenic regions, proliferating neural precursor cells and PSA+ postmitotic cells were found to form clusters. At times, the PSA+ cells were observed to give rise to short or long processes that surround BrdU-labeled newly generated cells (Seki 2002b). GFAP+ cells also engulf neighboring neuroblasts (Seki 2002b; Seri et al. 2004; Shapiro et al. 2005). Additionally, it has been proposed that neuronal, glial, and endothelial precursors divide in tight clusters that are located at a branch or terminus of fine capillaries, suggesting a vascular niche for adult hippocampal neurogenesis (Palmer et al. 2000). These observations show that in the neurogenic region of the adult hippocampus, various types of cells have intercellular relationships in a small area that may serve as an appropriate niche to support cell proliferation and differentiation of the neuronal precursors. In fact, GFAP+ cells from the adult hippocampus, but not the adult spinal cord, are reported to stimulate the proliferation of adult neural stem cells and the neural fate commitment in vitro (Song et al. 2002). It has also been proposed that endothelial cells stimulate the self-renewal of neural stem cells and the production of neurons (Shen et al. 2004). Whether or not neuroblasts or immature neurons play any role in cell proliferation and differentiation of neural progenitor cells in the adult hippocampus remains a subject of future investigation.

3 Migration and intercellular relationship

We have demonstrated that the subpopulation of PSA+ immature neurons or neuroblasts have tangential processes or basal dendrites (Seki 2002b). Furthermore, several reports have described immature granule cells with long tangential processes in the adult dentate granule cell layer of rats (Nacher et al. 2001; Seki 2002b; Seri et al. 2004; Esposito et al. 2005; Shapiro and Ribak 2005). Electrophysiological studies have revealed the presence of proliferative precursor cells with short tangential processes (van Praag et al. 2002; Fukuda et al. 2003; Kempermann et al. 2004; Esposito et al. 2005).

In addition, we have found that proliferating cells inside clusters develop short tangential processes, and when postmitotic cells withdraw from the proliferative site, they migrate tangentially and extend these tangential processes (unpublished data). Thereafter, the tangential processes shorten and thin radial processes extend and become apical dendritic processes.

During the tangential migration, the migrating cells appeared to leave a tangential process behind in the clusters (Seki 2002b: unpublished data).

Although we do not know the specific function of the intercellular association between proliferating cells and migrating neuroblasts, it is worth noting that similar intercellular relationships have so far been well studied in the developing brain. The most well-known interaction is the migration of neuroblasts along radial glial processes in the developing neocortex (Rakic 1971). Recently it was demonstrated that the radial glial cells are neural progenitor cells (Miyata et al. 2001; Noctor et al. 2001; Tamamaki et al. 2001), which also means that proliferative neural progenitor cells and migrating neuroblasts make contact with each other. Taken together, these results suggest that embryonic and adult neurogenesis share similar mechanisms in the intercellular relationships between proliferating cells and migrating neuroblasts and that the intercellular association may play an important role in the proliferation and differentiation of neural precursor cells. To explain the function of intercellular apposition in the developing neocortex, it has been proposed that migrating neuroblasts express Delta and Neuregulin, and activate the Notch and ErbB pathways of proliferative neural progenitor cells or radial glia (Ever and Gaiano 2005). However, it remains to be investigated what developmental signals function in adult hippocampal neurogenesis.

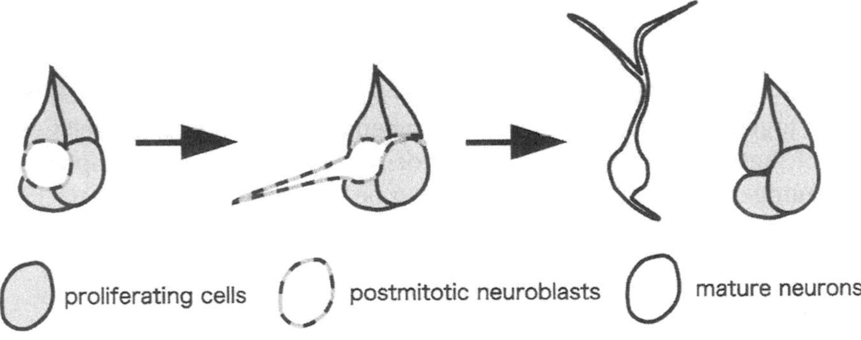

Fig. 2. Clustering, tangential migration and neurite formation of newly generated cells in the adult hippocampus. Proliferating cells and postmitotic neuroblasts make a cluster. When the postmitotic neuroblasts withdraw from the cluster, they move tangentially, extending tangentially oriented processes, one of whose processes is left behind within the cluster. Then the neuroblasts extend an apical process that finally becomes apical dendrites of the granule cell.

4 Adult neurogenesis and regenerative medicine

Neurogenesis in the adult brain suggests the possibility that adult neural tissue can regenerate after brain trauma. Actually, brain damage such as epilepsy and ischemia have been shown to up-regulate the production of new granule neurons, although it is unknown whether or not the new neurons restore the damaged brain tissue. There are two strategies for regenerative medicine of brain tissue: transplantation of neural stem cells and activation of intrinsic adult neurogenesis. However, transplantation experiments indicate that when neural stem or progenitor cells from neurogenic regions are transplanted into non-neurogenic regions, such as the cerebellum and spinal cord, they differentiate only into glia (Suhonen et al. 1996; Shihabuddin et al. 2000), although they develop into neurons if they are transplanted into neurogenic regions, such as the hippocampus and olfactory bulb. This suggests that the neurogenic regions possess special microenvironments to support neuronal differentiation. Astrocytes, postmitotic neuroblasts and blood vessels have been proposed as candidates of the microenvironments (Palmer et al. 2000; Seki 2002b). As mentioned above, these cells have a close intercellular relationship with proliferative neural progenitors. Furthermore, the findings of several *in vitro* experiments suggest that astrocytes and blood vessels release factors that regulate proliferation and differentiation of neural progenitor cells (Song et al. 2002; Shen et al. 2004). Additionally, GABAergic interneurons are reported to regulate the differentiation of the neural precursors (Tozuka et al. 2005). Taken together, systematic cellular arrangement and intercellular relationship of these cells could serve as microenvironments for adult hippocampal neurogenesis. However, it remains to be studied if and how these microenvironments play any role in the regeneration of brain tissue.

References

Altman J, Das GD (1965) Autoradiographic and histological evidence of postnatal hippocampal neurogenesis in rats. J Comp Neurol 124: 319-335.

Doetsch F, Caille I, Lim DA, Garcia-Verdugo JM, Alvarez-Buylla A (1999) Subventricular zone astrocytes are neural stem cells in the adult mammalian brain. Cell 97: 703-716.

Esposito MS, Piatti VC, Laplagne DA, Morgenstern NA, Ferrari CC, Pitossi FJ, Schinder AF (2005) Neuronal differentiation in the adult hippocampus recapitulates embryonic development. J Neurosci 25: 10074-10086

Ever L, Gaiano N (2005) Radial 'glial' progenitors: neurogenesis and signaling. Curr Opin Neurobiol 15: 29-33

Filippov V, Kronenberg G, Pivneva T, Reuter K, Steiner B, Wang LP, Yamaguchi M, Kettenmann H, Kempermann G (2003) Subpopulation of nestin-expressing progenitor cells in the adult murine hippocampus shows electrophysiological and morphological characteristics of astrocytes. Mol Cell Neurosci 23: 373-382

Fukuda S, Kato F, Tozuka Y, Yamaguchi M, Miyamoto Y, Hisatsune T (2003) Two distinct subpopulations of nestin-positive cells in adult mouse dentate gyrus. J Neurosci 23: 9357-9366

Goldman SA, Nottbohm F (1983) Neuronal production, migration, and differentiation in a vocal control nucleus of the adult female canary brain. Proc. Natl. Acad. Sci. USA 80: 2390-2394

Gould E, Cameron HA, Daniels DC, Woolley CS, McEwen BS (1992) Adrenal hormones suppress cell division in the adult rat dentate gyrus. J Neurosci 12: 3642-3650.

Gould E, Gross CG (2002) Neurogenesis in adult mammals: some progress and problems. J Neurosci 22: 619-623.

Kaplan MS (2001) Environment complexity stimulates visual cortex neurogenesis: death of a dogma and a research career. Trends Neurosci 24: 617-620.

Kaplan MS, Hinds JW (1977) Neurogenesis in the adult rat: electron microscopic analysis of light radioautographs. Science 197: 1092-1094

Kempermann G, Jessberger S, Steiner B, Kronenberg G (2004) Milestones of neuronal development in the adult hippocampus. Trends Neurosci 27: 447-452

Kuhn HG, Dickinson-Anson H, Gage FH (1996) Neurogenesis in the dentate gyrus of the adult rat: age-related decrease of neuronal progenitor proliferation. J Neurosci 16: 2027-2033

Miller MW, Nowakowski RS (1988) Use of bromodeoxyuridine-immunohistochemistry to examine the proliferation, migration and time of origin of cells in the central nervous system. Brain Res 457: 44-52

Miyata T, Kawaguchi A, Okano H, Ogawa M (2001) Asymmetric inheritance of radial glial fibers by cortical neurons. Neuron 31: 727-741.

Nacher J, Crespo C, McEwen BS (2001) Doublecortin expression in the adult rat telencephalon. Eur J Neurosci 14: 629-644.

Noctor SC, Flint AC, Weissman TA, Dammerman RS, Kriegstein AR (2001) Neurons derived from radial glial cells establish radial units in neocortex. Nature 409: 714-720.

Palmer TD, Willhoite AR, Gage FH (2000) Vascular niche for adult hippocampal neurogenesis. J Comp Neurol 425: 479-494

Rakic P (1971) Guidance of neurons migrating to the fetal monkey neocortex. Brain Res 33: 471-476

Seaberg RM, van Der Kooy D (2002) Adult rodent neurogenic regions: the ventricular subependyma contains neural stem cells, but the dentate gyrus contains restricted progenitors. J Neurosci 22: 1784-1793.

Seki T (2002a) Expression patterns of immature neuronal markers PSA-NCAM, CRMP-4 and NeuroD in the hippocampus of young adult and aged rodents. J Neurosci Res 70: 327-334

120

Seki T (2002b) Hippocampal adult neurogenesis occurs in a microenvironment provided by PSA-NCAM-expressing immature neurons. J Neurosci Res 69: 772-783.

Seki T, Arai Y (1991) The persistent expression of a highly polysialylated NCAM in the dentate gyrus of the adult rat. Neurosci Res 12: 503-513

Seki T, Arai Y (1993) Highly polysialylated neural cell adhesion molecule (NCAM-H) is expressed by newly generated granule cells in the dentate gyrus of the adult rat. J Neurosci 13: 2351-2358

Seki T, Arai Y (1995) Age-related production of new granule cells in the adult dentate gyrus. Neuroreport 6: 2479-2482

Seri B, Garcia-Verdugo JM, Collado-Morente L, McEwen BS, Alvarez-Buylla A (2004) Cell types, lineage, and architecture of the germinal zone in the adult dentate gyrus. J Comp Neurol 478: 359-378

Seri B, Garcia-Verdugo JM, McEwen BS, Alvarez-Buylla A (2001) Astrocytes give rise to new neurons in the adult mammalian hippocampus. J Neurosci 21: 7153-7160.

Shapiro LA, Korn MJ, Shan Z, Ribak CE (2005) GFAP-expressing radial glia-like cell bodies are involved in a one-to-one relationship with doublecortin-immunolabeled newborn neurons in the adult dentate gyrus. Brain Res 1040: 81-91

Shapiro LA, Ribak CE (2005) Integration of newly born dentate granule cells into adult brains: hypotheses based on normal and epileptic rodents. Brain Res Brain Res Rev 48: 43-56

Shen Q, Goderie SK, Jin L, Karanth N, Sun Y, Abramova N, Vincent P, Pumiglia K, Temple S (2004) Endothelial cells stimulate self-renewal and expand neurogenesis of neural stem cells. Science 304: 1338-1340

Shihabuddin LS, Horner PJ, Ray J, Gage FH (2000) Adult spinal cord stem cells generate neurons after transplantation in the adult dentate gyrus. J Neurosci 20: 8727-8735.

Song H, Stevens CF, Gage FH (2002) Astroglia induce neurogenesis from adult neural stem cells. Nature 417: 39-44.

Suhonen JO, Peterson DA, Ray J, Gage FH (1996) Differentiation of adult hippocampus-derived progenitors into olfactory neurons in vivo. Nature 383: 624-627

Tamamaki N, Nakamura K, Okamoto K, Kaneko T (2001) Radial glia is a progenitor of neocortical neurons in the developing cerebral cortex. Neurosci Res 41: 51-60.

Tozuka Y, Fukuda S, Namba T, Seki T, Hisatsune T (2005) GABAergic excitation promotes neuronal differentiation in adult hippocampal progenitor cells. Neuron 47: 803-815

van Praag H, Schinder AF, Christie BR, Toni N, Palmer TD, Gage FH (2002) Functional neurogenesis in the adult hippocampus. Nature 415: 1030-1034.

Involvement of β Isoform of PKC in PACAP-induced Differentiation of Neural Stem Cells into Astrocytes

Shigeo Nakajo[1], Jun Watanabe[2,3], Motoi Ohba[4], Fusako Ohno[1], Sakae Kikuyama[3], Kazuyasu Nakaya[5], and Seiji Shioda[2]

[1]Laboratory of Biological Chemistry, School of Pharmaceutical Sciences, Showa University, 1-5-8 Hatanodai, Shinagawa-ku, Tokyo 142-8555, Japan,
[2]Department of First Anatomy, School of Medicine, Showa University, 1-5-8 Hatanodai, Shinagawa-ku, Tokyo 142-8555, Japan
[3] Department of Biology, School of Education, Waseda University, 1-6-1 Nishi-Waseda, Shinjuku-ku, Tokyo 169-8050, Japan
[4] Institute of Molecular Oncology, Showa University, 1-5-8 Hatanodai, Shinagawa-ku, Tokyo 142-8555, Japan
[5] Faculty of Applied Life Sciences, Niigata University of Pharmacy and Applied Life Sciences, Niigata 956-8603, Japan
[1]Present address: Laboratory of Biochemistry, Yokohama College of Pharmacy, 601 Matanocyo, Totsuka-ku, Yokohama 245-0066, Japan

Summary. We have found that pituitary adenylate cyclase-activating polypeptide (PACAP) induces the differentiation of mouse neural stem cells (NSCs) into astrocytes via a mechanism that is independent of the cyclic AMP/protein kinase A pathway. NSCs expressed PACAP receptor, PAC1 on the plasma membranes. PACAP-induced differentiation was inhibited by the most potent antagosist, the phospholipase C (PLC) inhibitor, the protein kinase C (PKC) inhibitor, and the intracellular calcium chelator, and was mimicked by phorbol ester (PMA). These results suggest that the PACAP-generated signal was mediated via the PACAP receptor, PAC1 stimulated heterotrimeric G-protein, resulting in activation of PLC, followed by conventional PKC (cPKC). Embryonic NSCs expressed α, βI and βII isoforms of cPKC , but lacked PKCγ. When NSCs were exposed to PACAP, protein expression levels of the βI and βII transiently increased prior to differentiation, returning to basal levels by day 4, whereas the level of PKCα increased linearly up to day 6. Overexpression of PKCβII synergistically enhanced differentiation in the presence of PACAP, whereas expression of the dominant-negative mutant of PKCβII proved inhibitory. These results indicate that the βI/βII isoforms of PKC play a crucial role in the PACAP-induced differentiation of mouse embryonic NSCs into astrocytes.

122

Key words. neural stem cell, protein kinase C, differentiation, astrocyte, pituitary adenylate cyclase-activating polypeptide

1 Introduction

Neural stem cells (NSCs) are characterized by their capacity for self-renewal (Gage et al. 1995; Kuhn and Svendsen 1999) and their ability to generate all major cell types of the central nervous system (CNS) (Lendahl et al. 1990; Reynolds and Weiss 1992). NSCs are found in the embryonic and newborn CNS, as well as in restricted regions of the adult mammalian CNS, including the subventricular zone (SVZ) and the dentate gyrus of the hippocampus (Weissman et al. 2001), from which they can migrate to their final destinations and differentiate into terminal function cells (Gage 2000). Although a number of cell-intrinsic mechanisms and cell-extrinsic factors have been implicated in this process (Anderson 2001), the molecular mechanism underlying NSC differentiation remains unclear.

Pituitary adenylata cyclase-activating polypeptide (PACAP), which was originally purified from ovine hypothalamus (Miyata et al. 1989), is a neuropeptide belonging to the secretin/glucagon/vasoactive intestinal peptide (VIP) family. The physiological functions of PACAP are diverse, as it is thought to act as a hormone, a neurohormone, a neurotransmitter, and a trophic factor (Vaudry et al. 2000), and is found in a wide variety of tissues, including both the CNS and peripheral tissues such as the adrenal gland (Arimura et al. 1991), parathyroid (Luts and Sundler 1994), endocrine pancreas (Arimura and Shioda 1995; Love and Szebeni 1999) and testis (Arimura et al. 1991; Shioda et al. 1994). Based on this, it has been proposed that PACAP is able to act in a tissue-specific manner through its various receptors, PAC1, VPAC1 and VPAC2 (Spengler et al. 1993; Chatterjee et al. 1996; Nicot and DiCicco-Bloom 2001; Vaudry et al., 2000). The PAC1 receptor shows highest affinity for PACAP, while the latter two receptors possess equal affinity for PACAP and VIP (Vaudry et al., 2000). It has been demonstrated that PACAP and its receptors are expressed in rodent neocortex and its growth zones during the embryonic and postnatal periods, and that PACAP is involved in mediating pleiotropic physiological functions, such as neural proliferation, phenotypic determination, differentiation, survival, and neuroprotection (Lu and DiCicco-Bloom, 1997; Waschek et al., 1998; Zupan et al., 1998; Hill et al. 1999; Sköglosa et al., 1999; Zhou et al., 1999; Hansel et al., 2001; Nicot and DiCicco-Bloom, 2001; Shioda et al., 2006).

It is well known that protein phosphorylation contributes to intracellular signal propagation via ligand and receptor interactions. PACAP has been shown to cause cAMP production, protein kinase C

(PKC) activation and calcium mobilization in association with activation of PACAP receptors (Vaudry et al., 2000). Recently it has been demonstrated that PACAP-induced differentiation of rat NSCs into astrocytes involves cAMP/ protein kinase A (PKA) signal propagation (Vallejo and Vallejo 2002) and that activation of the phospholipase C (PLC) /PKC pathway is involved in the neuregulin-induced proliferation of hippocampus-derived nestin-expressing neural progenitor cells (Lai and Feng 2004). In addition, PACAP acting via the PAC1 receptor promotes the proliferation of NSCs in adult mouse brain. These findings have raised the possibility that PKC signaling is involved in mediating the effects of PACAP (Mercer et al. 2004). Thus it has variously been suggested that both PKA and PKC are involved in signal propagation leading to the proliferation or differentiation of neural progenitor cells. However, the precise molecular mechanism is not fully understood.

Previously we have shown that PACAP activates PKA, PKC, and calcium signaling cascades in rat neuroepithelial cells (Zhou et al., 2001), and promotes differentiation of embryonic NSCs into astrocytes through the PACAP receptor, PAC1 (Ohno et al., 2005). Here we describe that the β isoform of PKC plays a crucial role in the PACAP-induced differentiation of embryonic NSCs into astrocytes.

2 PACAP in Differentiation of NSCs

When isolated cells prepared from telencephalons of mouse E14.5 were cultured with bFGF, cells proliferated in a time-dependent manner. It has been showed that approximately 85% of the proliferating cells were immunopositive to monoclonal antibody against nestin. Furthermore, in the absence of bFGF, these cells differentiated into neurons, astrocytes, and oligodendrocytes following the addition of platelet-derived growth factor, ciliary neurotrophic factor (CNTF), and thyroid hormone T3, respectively, as described previously (Johe et al. 1996). The cells prepared in these experiments were characterized by self-renewing and multiple-lineage properties, indicating that they were NSCs.

During the exposure of NSCs to various substances in attempt to seek a novel differentiation factor, we found that morphological changes in these cells were evoked by PACAP at physiological concentations. To identify the cell types present, immunofluorescence staining using specific antibodies was performed. The results indicated that PACAP induced an increase in the number of GFAP-positive cells, which was significant at PACAP concentrations as well as 0.2 nM and maximal at 2 nM PACAP (Watanabe et al. 2006b). Approximately 55%, 30%, and 16% of cells reacted with 2 nM PACAP for 7 days were immunoreacted with antibodies against GFAP, nestin, and MAP-2, respectively, while anti-GalC immunoreactive cells accounted for just 4% of all cells. The

124

number of GFAP-positive cells increased about 6-fold in the presence of PACAP. This suggest that PACAP promotes proliferation of NSCs with increasing induction of differentiation. Coupled with the recent report that PACAP promotes NSCs proliferation in adult mouse brain (Mercer et al. 2004), these results are noteworthy for their demonstration of a new function for PACAP. Furthermore, the increase in the number of GFAP-positive cells was significantly antagonized by the addition of the most potent antagonist, $PACAP_{6-38}$. These results suggest that PACAP mainly induces the differentiation of NSCs into astrocytes via PACAP receptor on the plasma membranes of NSCs.

Given that PACAP induces the differentiation of mouse embryonic NSCs into astrocytes, it would therefore be necessary that peptide exists in the mouse embryonic brain. To this extent, radioimmunoassay experiments have shown that PACAP is present in rat brain at E14 (Tatsuno et al. 1994) and is widely expressed in the mouse neural tube at E10.5 (Waschek et al. 1996). However, it remains to be determined whether PACAP itself is expressed in embryo or transported from the maternal plasma across the placental barrier in the same manner as that for insulin-like growth factor and epidermal growth factor (Garnica and Chan 1996). Further experiments are needed to clarify the *in vivo* role of PACAP in the differentiation of NSCs into astrocytes.

3 Signal Transduction in PACAP-induced Differentiation

3.1 PACAP receptor and phospholipase C

Signal propagation in the differentiation process of NSCs by PACAP was investigated. First, expression of PACAP receptor in NSCs was evaluated. Three types of receptor, PAC1, VPAC1, and VPAC2, are well known to mediate the action of PACAP (Spengler et al. 1993, Chatterjee et al. 1996, Nicot and DiCicco-Bloom 2001). Among them, gene and its translational product of PACAP receptor, PAC1 that possesses the highest affinity for PACAP, were shown to be expressed on the plasma membrane of NSCs by RT-PCR and immunoblot analysis. Especially, a major band with apparent molecular weight of 53,000 was determined by immunoblot analysis. This is the first report which describes the expression of PACAP receptor protein in mouse NSCs (Ohno et al. 2005). PACAP-induced differentiation was significantly inhibited by the most potent antagosist, $PACAP_{6-38}$, as mentioned above. Therefore, it was thought PACAP acts on the PAC1 receptor on the plasma membranes of mouse NSCs.

We subsequently examined whether cyclic AMP (cAMP) plays an important role in the differentiation of NSCs by PACAP. NSCs were exposed to cAMP analogues such as 8Br-cAMP or dibutylic cAMP, with neither of these compounds inducing any change in the cells. In addition, the PACAP-induced differentiation and proliferation of NSCs could not be blocked by the protein kinase A (PKA) inhibitor, Rp-cAMP (Ohno et al. 2005). It has been reported that PACAP induces differentiation of rat cortical precursor cells into astrocytes (Vallejo and Vallejo 2002). They have also demonstrated that elevation of intracellular cAMP is responsible for the differentiation of cortical precursor cells into astrocytes since the induction by PACAP was influenced by a cAMP analogue and a PKA inhibitor. The discrepancy in the findings of these two studies might be due to differences in PACAP concentrations to which cells were exposed or species differences in the NSCs used in experiments.

We showed that neither cAMP analogues nor a PKA inhibitor had any effect on the differentiation of NSCs into astrocytes as described above, suggesting a signaling pathway that involves other receptor-coupled G protein rather than Gs. To ascertain whether the differentiation required activation of phospholipase C (PLC), the embryonic NSCs were exposed to a specific PLC inhibitor, U73122 at concentrations of 1-10 μM, 1 hr prior to the addition of PACAP. However, U73122 proved toxic even at the lowest concentration tested, requiring us to reduce the inhibitor concentration still further to 0.5 μM, despite the fact that U73122 is frequently used experimentally at a concentration of 10 μM. At 0.5 μM, U73122 led to 25% inhibition in the PACAP-induced NSC differentiation, suggesting that activation of PLC is a necessary step in this process. The PACAP receptor, PAC1, is a G protein-coupled receptor (GPCR) (Arimura 1998; Spengler 1993). It has been demonstrated that about 40% of all GPCRs utilize Gqα family members to stimulate inositol lipid signaling (Alexander and Peters 2000), and that PACAP activates the PLC signaling pathway, increasing intracellular calcium and eliciting translocation of PKC (Nicot and DiCicco-Bloom, 2001). Therefore, it is likely that PAC1 associates with the Gq class of heterotrimeric G proteins whose downstream effector is PLCβ (Hubbard and Hepler 2006). Thus PLC is thought to play a pivotal role downstream of the PAC1/Gq complex in the propagation of the differentiation signal induced by PACAP. The activation of PLC results in hydrolysis of phosphatidylinositol-4, 5-bisphosphate (PIP$_2$), leading to the production of diacylglycerol (DAG) and inositol 1,4,5-trisphosphate (IP$_3$) (Rhee 2001). IP$_3$ stimulates calcium mobilization and release of calcium from IP$_3$-regulated intracellular calcium stores, and both second messengers contribute to the activation of cPKC (Berridge 1987; Kikkawa et al. 1989).

3.2 Involvement of cPKC

We next examined the involvement of PKC, a molecule downstream of PLC. The effect of the benzophenanthridine alkaloid chelerythrine, an inhibitor of PKC (Herbert et al. 1990), was investigated, resulting in a

50% reduction in the number of astrocytes to almost basal levels. In addition, approximately 60% of the population expressed MAP2, similar to the percentage observed in the control experiment. Virtually, no cells were found to express the oligodendrocytic marker Gal-C.

When NSCs were exposed to PMA, a potent PKC activator, for 8 days in the absence of bFGF, the percentage of GFAP-immunopositive cells was 91% of that observed with PACAP alone, whereas 4α-PMA, an inactive analogue of PMA, had no effect. In order to ascertain whether the differentiation process was calcium dependent, the effect of an intracellular calcium chelator, BAPTA-AM, was examined. In the presence of BAPTA-AM, the number of GFAP-positive cells decreased by 40%, indicating that PACAP-induced differentiation was being significantly inhibited by the chelation of calcium. Although the PKC family is known to comprise at least 10 isoforms (Nishizuka 1995), these results were suspected to reflect the activation of Ca^{2+}- and phospholipid-dependent PKC, namely conventional PKC (cPKC), during the differentiation process.

3.3 Expression of cPKCs in embryonic NSCs

The isoforms of cPKC can be classified into three groups: PKCα, PKCβ (I and II) and PKCγ (Ohno et al. 1987; Yoshida et al. 1988; Nishizuka 1995). The regulatory domain of cPKC comprises two conserved membrane-targeting domains, C1 and C2, the former of which is known as a high-affinity receptor for DAG and phorbol esters, while the latter is able to bind calcium (Nishizuka, 1988; Ono et al., 1989; Irie et al. 2002). We investigated which subtypes of cPKC are expressed in embryonic NSCs based on their gene and protein expressions. Expression of the genes coding for the cPKC isoforms was assessed by RT-PCR, revealing that the genes coding for PKCα and PKCβI/II were expressed in NSCs as well as in adult cerebral cortex, while the gene coding for PKCγ was absent. It was shown that isoforms of cPKCs, PKCα and PKCβI/II were also detected by immunoblot analysis in embryonic NSCs. No immunoreactivity of PKCγ was revealed in those cells. In this study, PKCα, PKCβI and PKCβII were all found to be expressed in mouse embryonic NSCs. It has previously been demonstrated that PKCβ has the splicing variants, PKCβI and PKCβII, and that the latter is the predominant form generated from the PKCβ gene (Oka et al. 2002). However, immunoblot analysis revealed that PKCβI in embryonic NSCs is almost equally expressed, based on calculation of IgG concentrations of antibodies used. In contrast, gene and protein expression for the γ isoform, which is specifically found in the CNS (Saito et al. 1988), was not observed, although immunoreactivity for PKCγ with a molecular mass of approximately 80 kDa was detected by immunoblot analysis in the cerebral cortex of adult mouse. Other studies have similarly reported that PKCγ is not detected either in embryonic (E14.5) mouse whole brain (Watanabe et al. 2006a), or in early postnatal rat brain (Hashimoto et al. 1988; Yoshida et al. 1988), where PKCγ activity only begins to increase gradually a week after birth.

Although the function of PKCγ is unclear, recent reports have demonstrated that mutation of this isoform may be involved in the etiology of spinocerebellar ataxia (Chen et al., 2003; Warrenburg et al. 2003; Yabe et al. 2003; Stevanin et al. 2004; Seki et al. 2005). In addition, a point mutation in the PKCγ gene may contribute to retinitis pigmentosa (Al-Maghtheh, M. et al. 2001) and Parkinsonian syndrome (Campbell et al. 1997; Campbell et al. 2000; Payne et al. 2000). Possible neuronal functions, including involvement in synaptic plasticity and memory via modulation of long-term potentiation and long-term depression, have also been proposed (Saito and Shirai 2002).

Next, protein expression levels of PKCα, PKCβI and PKCβII during PACAP-induced differentiation of NSCs were investigated. PKCα expression increased linearly up to day 6, whereas PKCβI and PKCβII underwent a transient, approximately 2.0-fold increase up to day 2, then returned to basal levels by day 4. Similar changes in cPKC isoform protein expression have also been found in NSCs treated with CNTF, another inducer known as astrocytes inducing factor in NSC differentiation (Johe et al. 1996), suggesting that we may have been observing a general astrocytic differentiation mechanism. The changes in protein level are not due to translocation of cPKC from the soluble fraction to the membranes (Kraft et al. 1982; Zalewski et al. 1988; Kiley and Jaken 1990; Mochly-Rosen et al. 1990), given that intact NSCs were solubilized with lysis buffer containing 1% Triton X-100.

When NSCs were exposed to PACAP, the number of GFAP-expressing cells increased in a time-dependent manner, reaching a plateau at day 6. Morphological changes were first observed around 4-5 days (Ohno et al. 2005), which corresponded to the threshold for a marked increase in GFAP expression. In contrast, the maximal biosynthesis of PKCβI and PKCβII occurred earlier, before either morphological changes or a rise in the number of GFAP-positive cells was noted (Scheme 1). These findings suggest that while cPKCα may be involved in the PACAP-induced differentiation of NSCs into astrocytes, the transient increase in PKCβI and PKCβII protein synthesis may provide a crucial trigger for differentiation downstream of PLC.

128

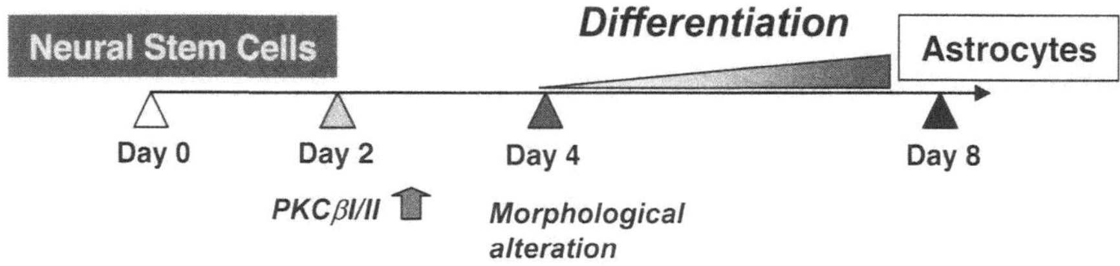

Scheme 1   Time course of PACAP-induced differentiation.

3.4 Responsibility of PKCβ for the PACAP-induced differerentiation

To verify the role of PKCα and PKCβII in the PACAP-induced differentiation of NSCs into astrocytes, the isoforms were overexpressed using an adenovirus (AdV) vector (Ohba et al. 1998; Berkner 1992). The isoform constructs were then introduced into embryonic NSCs, and protein expression levels evaluated by immunoblot analysis 2 days after virus infection. The results revealed strong expression compared with vehicle. Next, the effect of overexpression of the cPKC isoforms on the differentiation of NSCs was investigated. NSCs were infected with the AdV vectors, cultured for 8 days in the absence of PACAP, then subjected to immunofluorescence staining to analyze the nature of the differentiation. Unexpectedly, no change was observed in the absence of PACAP. However, the addition of 1 nM PACAP in association with overexpression of PKCβII synergistically caused the differentiation of NSCs into astrocytes, while in the case of PKCα the effect was additive. These results suggested that PACAP-induced differentiation requires the signaling pathways involving biosynthesis of either PKCα or PKCβII, or both, and triggering of their enzyme activities.

To further investigate the possible roles of PKCα and PKCβII, the effect of their dominant-negative mutants, KN-PKCα and KN-PKCβII, was determined. The results revealed that KN-PKCβII but not KN-PKCα significantly inhibits the PACAP-induced differentiation of embryonic NSCs into astrocytes, indicating that at least the βII isoform of cPKC is involved in the differentiation process.

The intracellular functions of PKC are diverse (Nishizuka 1988; Nishizuka 1992; Nishizuka 1995; Saito and Shirai 2002). Recently it has been demonstrated that PACAP acting via the PAC1 receptor promotes the proliferation of NSCs in adult mouse brain (Mercer et al. 2004), with the PKC inhibitor Gö6976 being used to demonstrate the involvement of PKC in this signaling pathway. In addition, proliferation of postnatal rat hippocampus neural progenitor cells, induced by neuregulin members of the EGF superfamily, via the PLC/PKC signaling pathway, has been reported (Lai and Feng 2004). However, as demonstrated in the present study, PKC also participates in the signal propagation driving differentiation of NSCs. It is possible that whether PKC signaling triggers proliferation or differentiation may be dependent on the subtypes and/or substrates of PKC expressed in the neural progenitor cells.

On the basis of data obtained thus far, we propose the following model of signal propagation in PACAP-induced differentiation of NSCs into astrocytes (Scheme 1): PACAP acts on the PAC1 receptor on the plasma membrane of NSCs, with the signal then being transmitted intracellularly via a PAC1-coupled G protein, which is probably $Gq\alpha$ heterotrimeric G protein. This leads to the activation of $PLC\beta$, followed by DAG and Ca^{2+} release from intracellular calcium stores by the action of IP_3, stimulating the $\beta I/II$ isoforms of cPKC. In addition, although the mechanism is not clear, this differentiation process also requires the transient biosynthesis of $PKC\beta I/II$, leading to differentiation into astrocytes via both signaling pathways. Further experiments are needed to clarify the substrate(s) of $PKC\beta$, which is thought to play a crucial role, and the molecular mechanism of gene regulation mediating its transient biosynthesis in the PACAP-induced differentiation of NSCs into astrocytes.

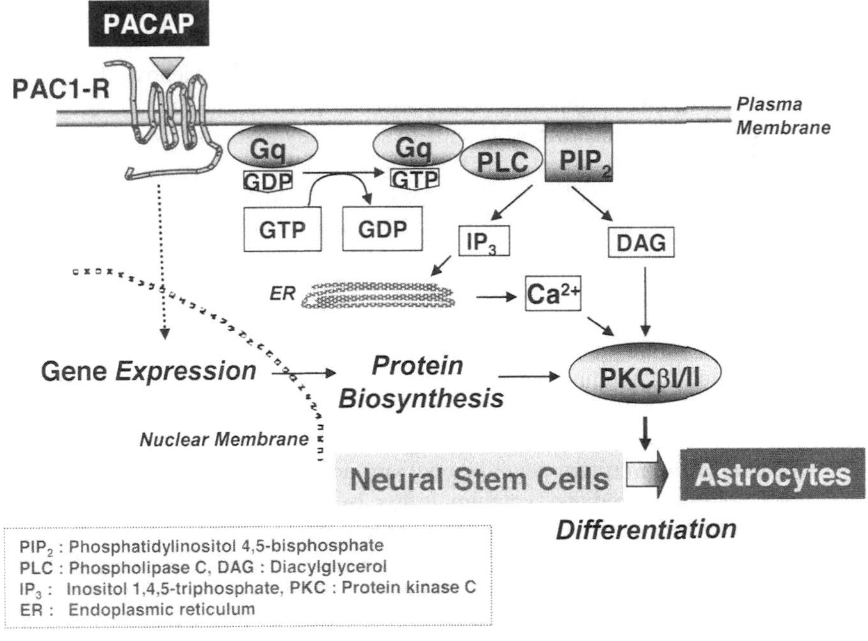

Scheme 2   Signal propagation of PACAP-induced differentiation in NSCs.

4 Acknowledgment

This work was supported in part by a Showa University Grant-in-Aid for Innovative Collaborative Research Projects.

References

Alexander SPH, Peters JA (Eds.) (2000) TiPS Receptor and Ion Channel Nomenclature Supplement. Elsevier.

Al-Maghtheh M, Vithana EN, Inglehearn CF, Moore T, Bird AC, Bhattacharya SS, (2001) A human homolog of yeast pre-mRNA splicing gene, PRP31, underlies autosomal dominant retinitis pigmentosa on chromosome 19q13.4 (RP11). Mol Cell 8:375-381

Anderson DJ (2001) Stem cells and pattern formation in the nervous system: the possible versus the actual. Neuron 30:19-35

Arimura A, Somogyvari-Vigh A, Miyata A, Mizuno K, Coy DH, Kitada C (1991) Tissue distribution of PACAP as determined by RIA: highly abundant in the rat brain and testes. Endocrinology 129:2787-2789

Arimura A, Shioda S (1995) Pituitary adenylate cyclase activating polypeptide (PACAP) and its receptors: neuroendocrine and endocrine interaction. Front. Neuroendocrinol 16:53-88

Arimura A (1998) Perspectives on pituitary adenylate cyclase activating polypeptide (PACAP) in the neuroendocrine, endocrine, and nervous systems. Jpn J Physiol 48:301-331

Berkner KL, (1992) Expression of heterologous sequences in adenoviral vectors. Curr Top Microbiol Immunol 158:39-66

Berridge MJ (1987) Inositol trisphosphate and diacylglycerol: two interacting second messengers. Annu Rev Biochem 56:159-193

Campbell JM, Payne AP, Gilmore DP, Russell D, McGadey J, Clarke DJ, Branton R, Davies RW, Sutcliffe RG (1997) Age changes in dopamine levels in the corpus striatum of Albino Swiss (AS) and AS/AGU mutant rats. Neurosci Lett 12:54-56

Campbell JM, Gilmore DP, Russell D, Growney CA, Favor G, Kennedy AK, Davies RW, Payne AP, Stone TW (2000) Pharmacological analysis of extracellular dopamine and metabolites in the striatum of conscious as/agu rats, mutants with locomotor disorder. Neuroscience 100:45-52

Chatterjee TK, Sharma RV, Fisher RA (1996) Molecular cloning of a novel variant of the pituitary adenylate cyclase-activating polypeptide (PACAP) receptor that stimulates calcium influx by activation of L-type calcium channels. J Biol Chem 271:32226-32232

Chen DH, Brkanac Z, Verlinde CL, Tan XJ, Bylenok L, Nochlin D, Matsushita M, Lipe H, Wolff J, Fernandez M, Cimino PJ, Bird TD, Raskind WH (2003) Missense mutations in the regulatory domain of PKC γ: a new mechanism for dominant nonepisodic cerebellar ataxia. Am J Hum Genet 72:839-849

Gage FH, Ray J, Fisher LJ (1995) Isolation, characterization, and use of stem cells from the CNS. Annu Rev Neurosci 18:159-192

Gage FH (2000) Mammalian neural stem cells. Science 287:1433-1438

Garnica AD, Chan WY (1996) The role of the placenta in fetal nutrition and growth. J Am Coll Nutr 15:206-222

Hansel DE, May V, Eipper BA, Ronnett GV (2001) Pituitary adenylyl cyclase-activating peptides and alpha-amidation in olfactory neurogenesis and neuronal survival in vitro. J Neurosci 21:4625-4636

Herbert JM, Augereau JM, Maffrand J.P (1990) Chelerythrine is a potent and specific inhibitor of protein kinase C. Biochem Biophys Res Commun 172:993-999.

Hill JM, Lee SJ, Dibbern DA Jr, Fridkin M, Gozes I, Brenneman DE (1999) Pharmacologically distinct vasoactive intestinal peptide binding sites: CNS localization and role in embryonic growth. Neuroscience 93:783-791

Hubbard KB, Hepler JR (2006) Cell signaling diversity of the Gqα family of heterotrimeric G proteins. Cell Signal 18:135-150

Irie K, Nakahara A, Nakagawa Y, Ohigashi H, Shindo M, Fukuda H, Konishi H, Kikkawa U, Kashiwagi K, Saito N (2002) Establishment of a binding assay for protein kinase C isozymes using synthetic C1 peptides and development of new medicinal leads with protein kinase C isozyme and C1 domain selectivity. Pharmacol Ther 93:271-281

Johe KK, Hazel TG, Muller T, Dugich-Djordjevic MM, McKay RD (1996) Single factors direct the differentiation of stem cells from the fetal and adult central nervous system. Genes Dev 10:3129-3140

Kikkawa U, Kishimoto A, Nishizuka Y (1989) The protein kinase C family: heterogeneity and its implications. Annu Rev Biochem 58:31-44

Kiley SC, Jaken S (1990) Activation of alpha-protein kinase C leads to association with detergent-insoluble components of GH4C1 cells. Mol Endocrinol 4:59-68

Kraft AS, Anderson WB, Cooper HL, Sando JJ (1982) Decrease in cytosolic calcium/phospholipid-dependent protein kinase activity following phorbol ester treatment of EL4 thymoma cells. J Biol Chem 257:13193-13196

Kuhn HG, Svendsen CN (1999) Origins, functions, and potential of adult neural stem cells. Bioessays 21:625-630

Lai C, Feng L (2004) Neuregulin induces proliferation of neural progenitor cells via PLC/PKC pathway. Biochem Biophys Res Commun 319:603-611

Lendahl U, Zimmerman LB, McKay RD (1990) CNS stem cells express a new class of intermediate filament protein. Cell 60:585-595

Love JA, Szebeni K (1999) Morphology and histochemistry of the rabbit pancreatic innervation. Pancreas 18:53-64

Lu N, DiCicco-Bloom E (1997) Pituitary adenylate cyclase-activating polypeptide is an autocrine inhibitor of mitosis in cultured cortical precursor cells. Proc Natl Acad Sci USA 94:3357-3362

Luts L, Sundler F (1994) Peptide-containing nerve fibers in the parathyroid glands of different species. Regul Pept 50: 147-158

Mercer A, Rönnholm H, Holmberg J, Lundh H, Heidrich J, Zachrisson O, Ossoinak A, Frisén J, Patrone C (2004) PACAP promotes neural stem cell proliferation in adult mouse brain. J Neurosci Res 76:205-215

Miyata A, Arimura A, Dahl RR, Minamino N, Uehara A, Jiang L, Culler MD, Coy DH (1989) Isolation of a novel 38 residue-hypothalamic polypeptide which stimulates adenylate cyclase in pituitary cells. Biochem Biophys Res Commun 164:567-574

Mochly-Rosen D, Henrich CJ, Cheever L, Khaner H, Simpson PC (1990) Cell Regul 1:693-706

Nicot A, Dicicco-Bloom EM (2001) Regulation of neuroblast mitosis is

132

determined by PACAP receptor isoform expression. Proc Natl Acad Sci USA 98:4758-4763

Nishizuka Y (1988) The molecular heterogeneity of protein kinase C and its implications for cellular regulation. Nature 334:661-665

Nishizuka Y. (1992) Intracellular signalling by hydrolysis of phospholipids and activation of protein kinase C. Science 258:607-614

Nishizuka Y. (1995) Protein kinase C and lipid signaling for sustained cellular responses. FASEB J 9:484-496

Ohba M, Ishino K, Kashiwagi M, Kawabe S, Chida K, Huh NH, Kuroki T (1998) Induction of differentiation in normal human keratinocytes by adenovirus-mediated introduction of the eta and delta isoforms of protein kinase C. Mol Cell Biol 18:5199-5207

Ohno F, Watanabe J, Sekihara H, Hirabayashi T, Arata S, Kikuyama S, Shioda S, Nakaya K, Nakajo S (2005) Pituitary adenylatecyclase-activating polypeptide promotes differentiation of mouse neural stem cells into astrocytes. Regul. Peptides 126:115-122

Ohno S, Kawasaki H, Imajoh S, Suzuki K, Inagaki M, Yokokura H, Sakoh T, Hidaka H (1987) Tissue-specific expression of three distinct types of rabbit protein kinase C. Nature 325:161-166

Oka M, Hitomi T, Okada T, Nakamura S, Nagai H, Ohba M, Kuroki T, Kikkawa U, Ichihashi M (2002) Dual regulation of phospholipase D1 by proteininase C α in vivo. Biochem Biophys Res Commun 294:1109-1113

Ono Y, Fujii T, Igarashi K, Kuno T, Tanaka C, Kikkawa U, Nishizuka Y (1989) Phorbol ester binding to protein kinase C requires a cysteine-rich zinc-finger-like sequence. Proc Natl Acad Sci USA 86:4868-4871

Payne AP, Campbell JM, Russell D, Favor G, Sutcliffe RG, Bennett NK, Davies RW, Stone TW (2000) The AS/AGU rat: a spontaneous model of disruption and degeneration in the nigrostriatal dopaminergic system. J Anat 196:629-33

Reynolds BA, Weiss S (1992) Generation of neurons and astrocytes from isolated cells of the adult mammalian central nervous system. Science 255:1707-1710

Rhee SG (2001) Regulation of phosphoinositide-specific phospholipase C. Annu Rev Biochem 70:281-312

Saito N, Kikkawa U, Nishizuka Y, Tanaka C (1988) Distribution of protein kinase C-like immunoreactive neurons in rat brain. J Neurosci 8:369-382

Saito N, Shirai Y (2002) Protein kinase Cγ (PKCγ) : function of neuron specific isotype. J Biochem (Tokyo) 132:683-687

Seki T, Adachi N, Ono Y, Mochizuki H, Hiramoto K, Amano T, Matsubayashi H, Matsumoto M, Kawakami H, Saito N, Sakai N (2005) Mutant protein kinase Cγ found in spinocerebellar ataxia type 14 is susceptible to aggregation and causes cell death. J Biol Chem 280:29096-29106

Shioda S, Legradi G, Leung WC, Nakajo S, Nakaya K, Arimura A (1994) Localization of pituitary adenylate cyclase-activating polypeptide and its messenger ribonucleic acid in the rat testis by light and electron microscopic immunocytochemistry and in situ hybridization. Endocrinology 135:818-825

Shioda S, Ohtaki H, Nakamachi T, Dohi K, Watanabe J, Nakajo S, Arata S, Kitamura S, Okuda H, Takenoya F, Kitamura Y (2006) Pleiotropic functions of PACAP in the CNS: Neuroprotection and Neurodevelopment. Ann NY Acad Sci in press

Sköglosa Y, Takei N, Lindholm D (1999) Distribution of pituitary adenylate cyclase activating polypeptide mRNA in the developing rat brain. Brain Res Mol Brain Res 65:1-13

Spengler D, Waeber C, Pantaloni C, Holsboer F, Bockaert J, Seeburg PH, Journot L (1993) Differential signal transduction by five splice variants of the PACAP receptor. Nature 365:170-175

Stevanin G, Hahn V, Lohmann E, Bouslam N, Gouttard M, Soumphonphakdy C, Welter ML, Ollagnon-Roman E, Lemainque A, Ruberg M, Brice A, Durr A (2004) Mutation in the catalytic domain of protein kinase C γ and extension of the phenotype associated with spinocerebellar ataxia type 14. Arch Neurol 61:1242-1248

Tastuno I, Somogyvari-Vigh A, Arimura A (1994) Developmental changes of pituitary adenylate cyclase activating polypeptide (PACAP) and its receptor in the rat brain. Peptides 15:55-60

Vallejo I, Vallejo M (2002) Pituitary adenylate cyclase-activating polypeptide induces astrocyte differentiation of precursor cells from developing cerebral cortex. Mol Cell Neurosci 21:671-683

Vaudry D, Gonzalez BJ, Basille M, Yon L, Fournier A, Vaudry H (2000) Pituitary adenylate cyclase-activating polypeptide and its receptors: from structure to functions. Pharmacol Rev 52:269-324

van de Warrenburg BP, Verbeek DS, Piersma SJ, Hennekam FA, Pearson PL, Knoers NV, Kremer HP, Sinke RJ (2003) Identification of a novel SCA14 mutation in a Dutch autosomal dominant cerebellar ataxia family. Neurology 61:1760-1765

Waschek JA, Casillas RA, Nguyen TB, DiCicco-Bloom EM, Carpenter EM, Rodriguez WI (1998) Neural tube expression of pituitary adenylate cyclase-activating peptide (PACAP) and receptor: potential role in patterning and neurogenesis. Proc Natl Acad Sci U S A 95:9602-9607

Waschek JA, Ellison J, Bravo DT, Handley V (1996) Embryonic expression of vasoactive intestinal peptide (VIP) and VIP receptor genes. J Neurochem 66:1762-1765

Watanabe J, Ohno F, Shioda S, Kikuyama S, Nakaya K, Nakajo S (2006a) Involvement of protein kinase C in the PACAP-induced differentiation of neural stem cells into astrocytes. Ann NY Acad Sci in press

Watanabe J, Shioda S, Kikuyama S, Nakaya K, Nakajo S (2006b) Differentiation of neural stem cells into astrocytes by low concentration of pituitary adenylate cyclase-activating polypeptide (PACAP). Springer-Verlag Tokyo, in press.

Weissman IL, Anderson DJ, Gage F (2001) Stem and progenitor cells: origins, phenotypes, lineage commitments, and transdifferentiations. Annu Rev Cell Dev Biol 17:387-403

Yabe I, Sasaki H, Chen DH, Raskind WH, Bird TD, Yamashita I, Tsuji S, Kikuchi S, Tashiro K (2003) Spinocerebellar ataxia type 14 caused by a mutation in protein kinase C γ. Arch Neurol 60:1749-1751

Yoshida Y, Huang FL, Nakabayashi H, Huang K-P (1988) Tissue distribution of and developmental expression of protein kinase C isozymes. J Biol Chem 263:9868-9873

Zalewski PD, Forbes IJ, Valente L, Apostolou S, Hurst NP (1988) Translocation of protein kinase C to a Triton-insoluble sub-cellular compartment induced by the lipophilic gold compound auranofin. Biochem Pharmacol 37:1415-1417

Zhou CJ, Shioda S, Shibanuma M, Nakajo S, Funahashi H, Nakai Y, Arimura A, Kikuyama S (1999) Pituitary adenylate cyclase-activating polypeptide receptors during development: expression in the rat embryo at primitive streak stage. Neuroscience 93:375-391

Zhou CJ, Yada T, Kohno D, Kikuyama S, Suzuki R, Mizushima H, Shioda S (2001) PACAP activates PKA, PKC and Ca^{2+} signaling cascades in rat neuroepithelial cells. Peptides 22:1111-1117

Zupan V, Hill JM, Brenneman DE, Gozes I, Fridkin M, Robberecht P, Evrard P, Gressens P (1998) Involvement of pituitary adenylate cyclase-activating polypeptide II vasoactive intestinal peptide 2 receptor in mouse neocortical astrocytogenesis. J Neurochem 70:2165-2173

Does PACAP have therapeutic potential in the field of neuroregenerative medicine?

Hirokazu Ohtaki[1], Tomoya Nakamachi[1], Jun Watanabe[1], Sachiko Yofu[1,3], Masaji Matsunaga[3], Ryosuke Matsuno[1], Kenji Dohi[1,2], and Seiji Shioda[1]

[1] Department of Anatomy, and [2] Emergency and Clinical Care Medicine Showa University School of Medicine, 1-5-8 Hatanodai, Shinagawa-ku Tokyo 142-8555, Japan. [3] Gene Trophology Research Institute, Tokyo, 130-0012, Japan.

Summary. The incidence of stroke is gradually increasing in the industrialized world, and is a major cause of long-lasting disability. Several different strategies have been investigated as a means of either preventing the occurrence of stroke or suppressing the subsequent enlargement of the infarct volume. However, due to the narrowness of the therapeutic time window, we are still far from achieving an effective response. One finding that has offered new hope is the discovery that neurogenesis, long regarded as an impossibility in the adult brain, does indeed occur. This raises the possibility that the damaged brain might in fact be able to recover as well as other tissues and organs. In this paper, we will review both existing and potential strategies for the treatment of cerebrovascular disease. In particular, we will focus on the prospects of pituitary adenylate cyclase-activating polypeptide (PACAP), a neuropeptide that has been shown to exert both neuroprotective and neurogenic effects.

Key words. stroke, PACAP, PACAP receptor, interleukin-6

1 Therapeutic target of cerebrovascular diseases

Cerebrovascular disease, including brain hemorrhage and infarction (stroke), is the third leading cause of death in the industrialized world. While the number of patients suffering from brain hemorrhage has decreased dramatically due to a decline in the level of dietary salt intake, the incidence of brain infarction is gradually increasing. This is largely attributable to recent changes in life-style, including factors such as higher fatty foods consumption, smoking, and increased stress. Even when the life of the patient is saved, infarction often leads long-lasting neurological deficits in learning, memory, and sensory and motor function (Haapaniemi et al. 1997, Hankey et al. 2006). Given the social and economic consequences of an ischemic event, considerable effort has been directed towards both preventing and treating stroke.

The first strategy in combating stroke involves "prevention of the occurrence". Lack of exercise, higher caloric intake, an unbalanced diet, and smoking are all contributory factors in diseases such as hypertension, diabetes, and hyperlipemia, which in turn are well known to augment the risk of infarction. It is not surprising, therefore, that a healthier life-style is often recommended as a first line of defence, reducing the need for clinical intervention.

The second strategy focused on "suppression of enlargement of the infarct volume". This includes the development of drugs and treatment strategies to extend the therapeutic time window during the acute periods. After brain ischemia, the tissues lose oxygen and ATP as energy, and are ensnared in irreversible necrotic changes (Ohtaki et al. 2005). The therapeutic time window represents the period during which cells and tissues retain the ability to recover from such damage. In the case of neuronal cell death this allows 3 hours following the onset of ischemia (Szabo et al. 2005, De Keyser et al. 2005). For nearly a decade, numerous animal and clinical studies have been devoted to understanding the mechanisms and factors regulating the induction and suppression of neuronal cell death, and many drugs targets and therapeutic strategies have been pursued. One noteworthy achievement has been the development of MCI-186 (radicut), a free radical scavenger, for the treatment of cerebrovascular diseases (Abe et al. 1998). However, the frequent delay in hospitalization and diagnosis of the infarction (usually of the order of 1 to 1.5 hours) still detracts from the clinical potential of such treatment.

This leads to the third target: "neuroregeneration". Given the long-held brief that neurons could not divide and proliferate in adult brain, and that damaged neurons and tissues were therefore incapable of recovery, neuroregeneration was never considered a viable possibility. Recently, however, neural stem cells (NSCs) capable of undergoing neurogenesis have been identified in the adult brain, both in the subventricular zone lining the lateral ventricles and in the subgranular zone of the dentate gyrus (Gage 2000, Eriksson et al. 1998). Furthermore, neurogenesis has been shown to increase in response to brain injury following ischemia (Arvidsson et al. 2002, Taguchi et al. 2004). This response is believed to be directly stimulated by the induction of activated astrocytes, and indirectly mediated via the generation of various factors, including nerve growth factor, brain-derived neurotrophic factor, fibroblast growth factor 2, vascular endothelium growth factor, and erythropoietin (Song et al. 2002, Lichtenwalner and Parent 2006). It is considered that the NSCs and the neurogenesis associated with astrocytes contribute to the repair of the injured brain after ischemia (Arvidsson et al. 2002). These finding have raised strong expectations that the damaged brain might in fact be capable of the same level of recovery as that observed in other tissues and organs. However, neurogenesis mediated by endogenous NSCs cannot fully compensate for the neural loss observed in ischemic insults. Therefore, transplantation of embryonic, neuronal and mesenchymal stem cells, which act as both a source of neurons and an activator of neurogenesis, has also attracted considerable attention as a relevant strategy in neuroregenerative medicine.

2 PACAP

2.1 What is PACAP?

PACAP was first isolated from ovine hypothalamus in 1989 by Arimura and his colleagues. PACAP, a member of the vasoactive intestinal polypeptide (VIP)/secretin/growth hormone releasing family of peptides, has an amino acid sequence that shows greatest similarity to that of VIP. PACAP and VIP, which have a number of functions in common, share three receptors: the PAC1-receptor (PAC1-R), and the VPAC1- and VPAC2-receptors (VPAC1-R and VPAC2-R, respectively). The neuroprotective signaling pathway of VIP is initiated through the VPAC1-R and the VPAC2-R. PACAP binds with VPAC1-R and VPAC2-R with almost the same affinity as VIP, but has a 1,000-fold higher affinity than VIP for its specific receptor PAC1-R.

PACAP exists in 38- and 27-amino acid amidated forms. PACAP38, which is found 10-fold higher levels in the body than PACAP27, is a pleiotropic neuroendocrine peptide that can function as a neurotransmitter, neuromodulator, neurotrophic factor, vasodilator, or non-cholinergic catecholamine secretagogue, as well as acting as a modulator of immune cells. PACAP has also been shown to exert both neuroprotective and cell differentiated effects (Arimura 1998).

138

2.2 Neuroprotective effect of PACAP

The neuroprotective effect of PACAP was initially reported in 1996 in a rat global ischemia model (Uchida et al. 1996). In this and subsequent studies, PACAP has been shown to prevent neuronal cell death at very low concentrations, with its intracerebroventricular infusion in the rat preventing neuronal loss in the hippocampus and decreasing the extent of infarction after global and focal ischemia (Uchida et al. 1996, Reglodi et al. 2000, 2002, Dohi et al. 2002) Given that PACAP can cross the blood-brain barrier via a saturable mechanism (Banks et al. 1993, 1996), its intravenous injection has also been demonstrated to be effective in preventing ischemic neuronal damage (Uchida et al. 1996, Reglodi et al. 2000).

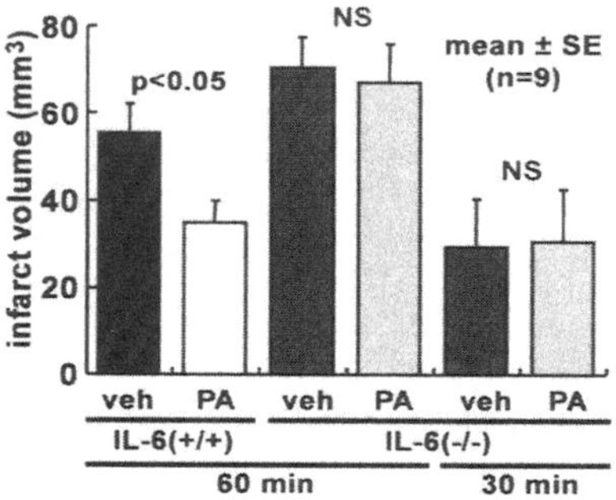

Fig. 1. The infarct volume in wild-type (IL-6$^{+/+}$) mice treated with PACAP is lower than that in animals treated with vehicle. In contrast, no PACAP-mediated neuroprotection is apparent in IL-6$^{-/-}$ mice following either 30 or 60 min transient focal ischemia.

Recently, we have demonstrated that PACAP decreases ischemic neuronal cell death in association with interleukin-6 (IL-6, see Fig. 1). PACAP and IL-6 regulate bcl-2, a known as an anti-apoptotic factor, and suppress cytochrome c release from mitochondria. Furthermore, using both PACAP and IL-6 null mice, we have shown that PACAP directly regulates the phosphorylation of extracellular-signal regulated kinase (ERK) while indirectly regulating signal transducer and activator of transcription 3 (STAT3) via the generation of IL-6 through PAC1-R in neurons (Fig. 2, Ohtaki et al. in press).

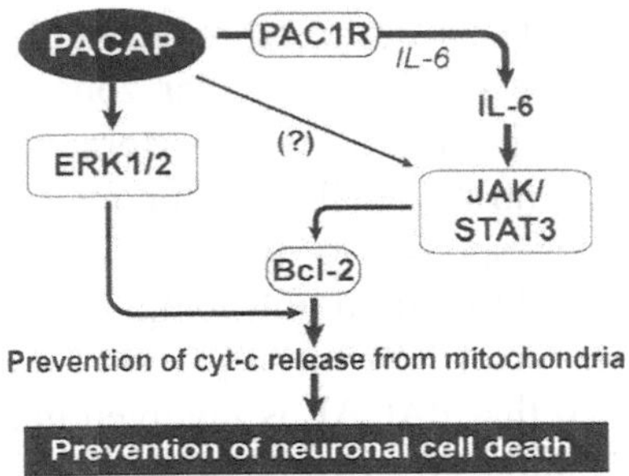

Fig. 2. Schematic diagram illustrating PACAP-mediated neuroprotection following ischemia.

2.3 Possibility of a role for PACAP in neuroregeneration

Various molecules, such as growth factors, have been reported to induce an increase in NSC proliferation and differentiation, but to date little attention has been focused on the effect of neuropeptides. Recently, however, some lines of evidence have led let us to speculate that PACAP might play a role in neurogenesis.

Using *in situ* hybridization, it has been shown that the PAC1-R gene is expressed in central nervous system of fetal rat during development (Zhou et al 1999, 2000), as well as in the subventricular zone lining the lateral ventricles and in the subgranular zone of the dentate gyrus of the adult mouse brain (Mercer et al. 2004). Both the gene and protein of PAC1R have also been detected in NSC primary culture form embryonic day 14.5 telencephalon, using RT-PCR and imunoblotting analyses (Ohno et al. 2004).

In cell culture studies, there is evidence to suggest that PACAP might be involved in neurogenesis. In PC12 cells, PACAP synergizes with NGF to stimulate PACAP gene transcription and neurite outgrowth, these being differentially dependent on the ERK1/2 and p38 MAP kinase pathways (Sakai et al. 2004). VIP and PACAP have also been shown to potently increase the proportion of ES cells expressing specifically expressing a neuronal phenotype, as revealed by immunocytochemistry and neurite outgrowth, without altering glial cell number (Cazillis et al. 2004). PACAP promotes NSC proliferation *in vitro* via PAC1-R and exerts a number of biological effects in addition to neurogenesis. It has been demonstrated that the molecular changes underlying the proliferative effects of PACAP are altered by the withdrawal of epidermal growth factor (EGF) in periventricular zone-derived adult NSC cultures (Sievertzon et al. 2005). The same authors also showed that intracerebroventricular infusion of PACAP increases cell proliferation in the ventricular zone of the lateral ventricle and the dentate gyrus of the hippocampus. Moreover, cultured NSCs isolated from the lateral ventricle wall of adult mice express PAC1-R and proliferate *in vitro* in response to two PAC1 agonists, PACAP and Maxadilan, but do respond to VIP at physiologic concentrations, indicating that PAC1-R is a mediator of NSC proliferation (Mercer et al. 2004). Recently, we have reported that PACAP is involved in inducing the differentiation of mouse NSCs into astrocytes (Ohno et al. 2005) and have demonstrated the presence of PAC1-R in the activated astrocytes (Suzuki et al. 2003).

This increasing body of evidence suggests that PACAP might regulate neurogenesis directly via stimulation of NSCs and indirectly via its effect on astrocytes.

5 Conclusions

The prospect of neruogeneration offers considerable hope as a new therapeutic strategy for cerebrovascular diseases. PACAP has been reported to play an important neuroprotective role following cerebral ischemia. Recently, evidence has been accumulating to suggest that PACAP might be involved in the regulation of neurogenesis. However, considerable work remains to be done before any therapeutic potential of these findings can be realized. Given that PACAP plays a unique role in both preventing neuronal cell death and accelerating neurogenesis via multiple pathways, we hope that future studies will continue to pursue an understanding of the underlying mechanisms, elucidating the best way in which the activity of PACAP can be harnessed for the treatment of cerebrovascular disease.

6 Acknowledgements

This work was supported in part by Showa University Grant-in Aid for Innovative Collaborative Research Projects (H.O) and Research on Health Sciences focusing on Drug Innovation from The Japan Health Sciences Foundation (S.S).

References

Abe K, Yuki S, Kogure K (1993) Strong attenuation of ischemic and postischemic brain edema in rats by a novel free radical scavenger. Stroke 19:480-485.

Arimura A (1998) Perspectives on pituitary adenylate cyclase activating polypeptide (PACAP) in the neuroendocrine, endocrine, and nervous systems. Jpn J Physiol 48:301-331

Arvidsson A, Collin T, Kirik D, Kokaia Z, Lindvall O (2002) Neuronal replacement from endogenous precursors in the adult brain after stroke. Nat Med 8:963-970

Banks WA, Kastin AJ, Komaki G, Arimura A (1993) Passage of pituitary adenylate cyclase activating polypeptide1-27 and pituitary adenylate cyclase activating polypeptide1-38 across the blood-brain barrier. J Pharmacol Exp Ther 267:690-696

Banks WA, Uchida D, Arimura A, Somogyvari-Vigh A, Shioda S (1996) Transport of pituitary adenylate cyclase-activating polypeptide across the blood-brain barrier and the prevention of ischemia-induced death of hippocampal neurons. Ann N Y Acad Sci 805:270-279

Cazillis M, Gonzalez BJ, Billardon C, Lombet A, Fraichard A, Samarut J, Gressens P, Vaudry H, Rostene W (2004) VIP and PACAP induce selective neuronal differentiation of mouse embryonic stem cells. Eur J Neurosci 19:798-808

De Keyser J, Uyttenboogaart M, Koch MW, Elting JW, Sulter G, Vroomen PC, Luijckx GJ (2005) Neuroprotection in acute ischemic stroke. Acta Neurol Belg 105:144-148

Dohi K, Mizushima H, Nakajo S, Ohtaki H, Matsunaga S, Aruga T, Shioda S (2002) Pituitary adenylate cyclase-activating polypeptide (PACAP) prevents hippocampal neurons from apoptosis by inhibiting JNK/SAPK and p38 signal transduction pathways. Regul Pept 109:83-88

Eriksson PS, Perfilieva E, Bjork-Eriksson T, Alborn AM, Nordborg C, Peterson DA, Gage FH (1998) Neurogenesis in the adult human hippocampus. Nat Med 4:1313-1317

Gage FH (2000) Mammalian neural stem cells. Science 287:1433–1438

Haapaniemi H, Hillbom M, Juvela S (1997) Lifestyle-associated risk factors for acute brain infarction among persons of working age. Stroke 28:26-30

Hankey GJ, Norman PE, Eikelboom JW (2006) Medical treatment of peripheral arterial disease. JAMA 295:547-553

Lichtenwalner RJ, Parent JM (2006) Adult neurogenesis and the ischemic forebrain. J Cereb Blood Flow Metab 26:1-20

Mercer A, Ronnholm H, Holmberg J, Lundh H, Heidrich J, Zachrisson O, Ossoinak A, Frisen J, Patrone C (2004) PACAP promotes neural stem cell proliferation in adult mouse brain. J Neurosci Res 76:205-215

Ohno F, Watanabe J, Sekihara H, Hirabayashi T, Arata S, Kikuyama S, Shioda S, Nakaya K, Nakajo S (2005) Pituitary adenylate cyclase-activating polypeptide promotes differentiation of mouse neural stem cells into astrocytes. Regul Pept 126:115-122

Ohtaki H, Dohi K, Nakamachi T, Yofu S, Endo S, Kudo Y, Shioda S (2005) Evaluation of brain ischemia in mice. Acta Histochem Cytochem 38:99-106.

Ohtaki H, Nakamachi T, Dohi K, Aizawa Y, Takaki A, Hodoyama K, Yofu S, Hashimoto H, Shintani N, Baba A, Kopf M, Iwakura Y, Matsuda M, Arimura A, Shioda S (2006) Pituitary adenylate cyclase-activating polypeptide (PACAP) decreases ischemic neuronal cell death in association with interleukin-6. Proc Natl Acad Sci USA (*in press*)

Reglodi D, Somogyvari-Vigh A, Vigh S, Kozicz T, Arimura A (2000) Delayed systemic administration of PACAP38 is neuroprotective in transient middle cerebral artery occlusion in the rat. Stroke 31:1411-1417

Reglodi D, Tamas A, Somogyvari-Vigh A, Szanto Z, Kertes E, Lenard L, Arimura A, Lengvari I (2002) Effects of pretreatment with PACAP on the infarct size and functional outcome in rat permanent focal cerebral ischemia. Peptides 23:2227-2234

Sakai Y, Hashimoto H, Shintani N, Katoh H, Negishi M, Kawaguchi C, Kasai A, Baba A (2004) PACAP activates Rac1 and synergizes with NGF to activate ERK1/2, thereby inducing neurite outgrowth in PC12 cells. Brain Res Mol Brain Res 123:18-26

Sievertzon M, Wirta V, Mercer A, Frisen J, Lundeberg J (2005) Epidermal growth factor (EGF) withdrawal masks gene expression differences in the study of pituitary adenylate cyclase-activating polypeptide (PACAP) activation of primary neural stem cell proliferation. BMC Neurosci 6:55

Song H, Stevens CF, Gage FH (2002) Astroglia induce neurogenesis from adult neural stem cells. Nature 417:39-44

Suzuki R, Arata S, Nakajo S, Ikenaka K, Kikuyama S, Shioda S (2003) Expression of the receptor for pituitary adenylate cyclase-activating polypeptide (PAC1-R) in reactive astrocytes. Brain Res Mol Brain Res 115:10-20

Szabo K, Lanczik O, Hennerici MG. (2005) Vascular diagnosis and acute stroke: what, when and why not? Cerebrovasc Dis 20 Suppl 2:11-8

Taguchi A, Soma T, Tanaka H, Kanda T, Nishimura H, Yoshikawa H, Tsukamoto Y, Iso H, Fujimori Y, Stern DM, Naritomi H, Matsuyama T (2004) Administration of CD34+ cells after stroke enhances neurogenesis via angiogenesis in a mouse model. J Clin Invest 114:330-338

Uchida D, Arimura A, Somogyvari-Vigh A, Shioda S, Banks WA (1996) Prevention of ischemia-induced death of hippocampal neurons by pituitary adenylate cyclase activating polypeptide. Brain Res 736:280-286

Zhou CJ, Kikuyama S, Nakajo S, Hirabayashi T, Mizushima H, Shioda S (2000) Splice variants of PAC1 receptor during early neural development of rats. Peptides 21:1177-1183

Zhou CJ, Shioda S, Shibanuma M, Nakajo S, Funahashi H, Nakai Y, Arimura A, Kikuyama S (1999) Pituitary adenylate cyclase-activating polypeptide receptors during development: expression in the rat embryo at primitive streak stage. Neuroscience 93:375-391

The Surgical Procedures of Hippocampal Ischemia Models for the Study of Regeneration in Rats

Kenji Dohi [1], Hirokazu Ohtaki[2], Yoshifumi Kudo[3], Tomoya Nakamachi[2], Seiji Shioda[2], Tohru Aruga[1]

[1]Department of Emergency and Critical Care Medicine, [2]Department of Anatomy I , [3]Department of Orthopedic Surgery, Showa University School of Medicine, 1-5-8 Hatanodai, Shinagawa-ku, Tokyo 142-8555, Japan

Summary. The pyramidal neurons of the hippocampal CA1 region are essential for cognitive functions such as spatial learning and memory, and are vulnerable to ischemic stress. Transient ischemic stress causes selective neuronal cell death in the CA1 region. Recently, it has been reported that degenerated CA1 pyramidal neurons recovered late after ischemia. Since this discovery, study of the regeneration of CA1 pyramidal neurons has increased. There are two types of ischemic model for animal research, the focal ischemic model and the global ischemic model. Global ischemic models are useful for the study of regeneration of CA1 pyramidal neurons. In this presentation, we introduced various rat global ischemic models for the study of regeneration of CA1 pyramidal neurons.

Key words. Regeneration, rat, global ischemia, neuronal cell death, CA1

1   Introduction

Neurons are vulnerable to various stresses such as heat stress, hypoxic stress, hypoglycemia, and ischemic stress. Hippocampal CA1 pyramidal neurons are especially vulnerable in comparison to other areas. They are destroyed by brief ischemia, but neuronal degeneration is not observed immediately after ischemia. Degeneration of pyramidal neurons progresses gradually from 4 days after ischemia, a phenomenon known as "delayed neuronal cell death (DND) (Kirino 1982, Dohi et al. 1998). Morphologically, DND is thought to be apoptosis and is characterized by fragmentation of the nucleus, cell shrinkage, and the disappearance of slight cilia on the cell surface. (Wyllie et al, 1980) At least three models of ischemia have been developed for the study of DND in the CA1 region of rats. These global ischemic models can be classified as applying to two types of ischemia, forebrain ischemia and whole body ischemia (Fig. 1). The forebrain ischemia models are the four-vessel occlusion model (4VO) (Kirino et al. 1982) and the two-vessel occlusion and hypotension model (2VO + H) (Koh et al. 1996, Hartman et al. 2005). The whole body ischemia model is the cardiac-arrest model.

The 4VO model causes a delayed neuronal cell death (Beilharz et al. 1995, MacManus et al. 1993, Nitatori et al. 1995), but the main defect of this model is a large inter-animal variability in the blockade of the cerebral circulation, which makes quantitative analysis of the ischemic effects very difficult. Also, this method is very invasive. The 2VO+H model of transient global ischemia produced significant damage to the dorsal hippocampal CA1 field in rats and is associated with impaired spatial learning in the absence of any other observable behavioral deficits studies. Compared to models in which vessels are permanently occluded, the transient occlusion used in this model more closely approximates an episode of transient forebrain hypoxic-ischemia in humans. Additionally, because the vascular system remains intact, 2VO + H is attractive for long-term studies of cognitive deficits and neurodegeneration following an ischemic event (Koh et al. 1996, Hartman et al. 2005).

The cardiac arrest model was developed to improve the shortcomings of the four-vessel occlusion model and is a sure way to achieve hemostasis, and this method is less invasive than other methods (Kawai et al. 1992, Korpatchev 1982, Dohi K et al. 1998). Recently, we developed a new whole body ischemia model (Kudo et al. 2006). The inductions of ischemia in this model are caused by drawing blood and compressing the heart. The ischemic insults are thus caused by cardiac arrest and hypotension (shock). Hippocampal CA1 pyramidal neurons and the spinal cord are also degenerated in this model. The surgical procedure of this model is not difficult, and it is less invasive than other methods. Moreover, the vascular system remains intact.

In this report, we introduce the surgical procedures of these models.

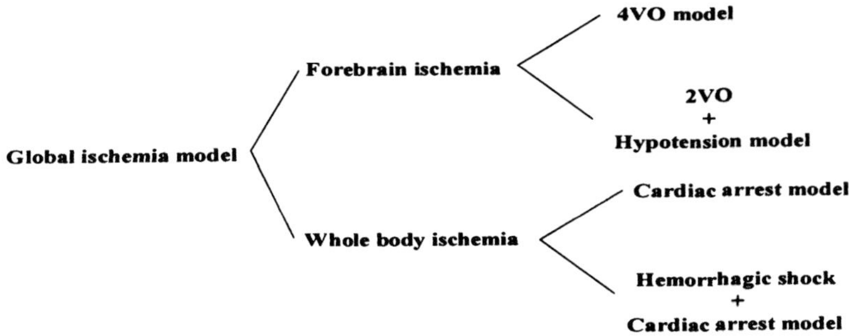

Fig. 1. The classification of rat global ischemia models.

2 The Surgical Procedures of the Forebrain Ischemic Model

2.1 Four vessels occlusion model (4VO) (Pulsinelli et al. 1979)

Male Wistar rats weighing between 250 and 300 g were anesthetized with ether and both common carotid arteries isolated via a ventral, midline cervical incision. An atraumatic arterial clasp was loosely placed around each common carotid artery without interrupting carotid blood flow, and the incision was closed with a single suture. A second incision, 1 cm long, was made behind the occipital bone directly overlying the first two cervical vertebrae. The paraspinal muscles were separated from the midline, and with the use of an operating microscope, the right and left alar foramina of the first cervical vertebrae and left alar foramina of the first vertebrae were exposed (Fig. 2). Various types of physiological monitoring were done (EEG, core temperature monitor, etc.). Each animal's core temperature was continuously monitored with a flexible rectal thermometer and maintained at 37°C. The awake rats were then held by hand in a simple restraint, the ventral neck suture was removed, and both carotid clasps were tightened to produce 4-vessel occlusion.

146

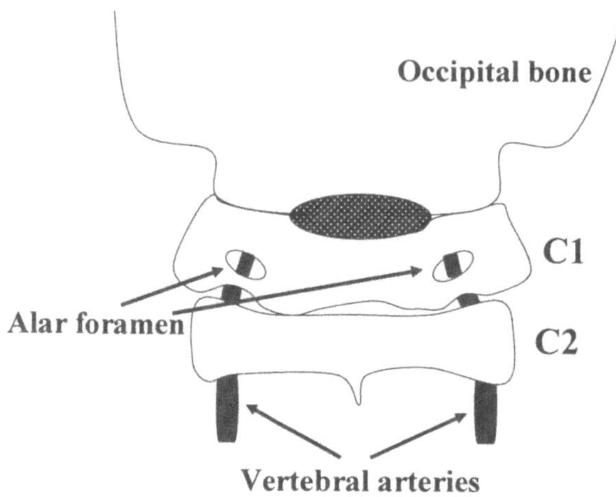

Fig. 2. The anatomical features of the 4-vessel occlusion model (4VO). Bilateral vertebral arteries were coagulated and occluded at the alar foramens.

2.2 Two-vessel occlusion and hypotension (2VO + H) (Koh et al. 1996)

Anesthesia was maintained with 1.5% halothane/27% O_2/balanced NO_2. For continuous monitoring of blood pressure, blood sampling, and induction of hemorrhagic hypotension during ischemia, the femoral arteries were cannulated bilaterally with polyethylene tubing (PE-50) and filled with 50 U/ml heparinised saline. Via a ventral midline neck incision, the common carotid arteries were exposed and silk thread with silastic tubing was placed loosely around the isolated arteries. Both cranial and rectal temperatures were measured via a thermocouple (Physitemp, New Jersey, USA) and were maintained at 37±0.2 °C with a heating fan and pad. A bipolar EEG was recorded using two active lateral electrodes and a reference central scalp electrode, which were interfaced with a bioamplifier. The EEG and arterial blood pressure were recorded. Plasma glucose levels were measured with a blood glucose meter.

Following a 10-min stabilization period, global ischemia was induced by occluding both common carotid arteries. Arterial blood was withdrawn to maintain a mean arterial blood pressure of 45 mm Hg. TGI was recorded from the time the EEG became isoelectric and was maintained for 8 min. At the completion of global ischemia, the carotid clamps were removed and the warmed blood reinfused. The animals were monitored post-ischemia for a period of 10 min with recording of arterial blood pressure, EEG, and temperature. At 10 min following removal of the carotid clamps the blood gas measurements were repeated. Arterial lines were then removed and the wounds sutured. The animals were extubated, allowed to recover, and returned to their cages with free access to food and water until being sacrificed 7 days later. Rectal temperature was monitored for 6 h post-surgery. Sham-operated animals received identical anesthesia and surgery as experimental animals but were not rendered ischemic.

3. The Surgical Procedures of Whole Body Ischemia

3.1 Cardiac arrest model (Korpatchev et al. 1982, Dohi et al. 1998)

The animals were intubated under anesthesia with 3.5% halothane and maintained with 2% sevoflurane in 70% N20 and 30% 02. Core temperature was continuously monitored with a flexible rectal thermometer and maintained at 37°C. A polyethylene catheter was inserted into the left femoral artery. Blood pressure and the electrocardiogram were monitored during all of the procedures. Global cerebral ischemia was induced according to the rat cardiac-arrest model. (Korpatchev et al. 1982, Kawai et al. 1992, Dohi et al. 1998) With the anesthetized rat in the supine position, an incision, about 0.5 cm in length, was made in the midline of the chest (Fig. 3A). The occluding device (Fig. 3B) was gently inserted in the mediastinum at the level of the second intercostal segment. The device was manipulated, with its distal end moved along the dorsal wall of the thorax. Then the distal end was twisted 45° in order to position it under the bundle of the superior aortic artery. A complete interruption of the circulation, due to compression of the superior aortic artery, was accomplished by lifting the occluding device and, at the same time, applying pressure with the fingers from outside (Fig. 3C). After 5 minutes of transient global ischemia, under artificial ventilation (100% O2), heart massage was then commenced in order to facilitate resuscitation. After a recovery period of 30 minutes, the animals could be disconnected from the respirator. The animals were housed in cages with free access to food

148

pellets and water. Fig. 4 shows regional cerebral blood flow and blood pressure during cardiac arrest and recirculation. The figure also shows the time course of the neurological parameters during the operation. The in situ terminal deoxynucleotidyl transferase-mediated dUTP nick-end labeling (TUNEL) method is shown in Fig. 5. Many TUNEL-positive pyramidal neurons were observed at 7 days after ischemia.

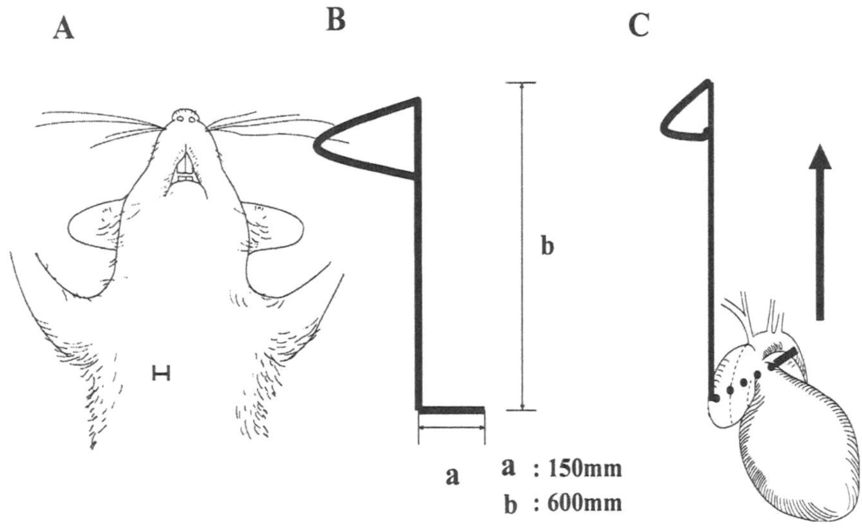

Fig. 3A, B, C. The surgical procedures and the occluding device of this model. Skin incision in this model (A). The scheme of the occluding device (B). Scheme of the surgical procedure(C). The major cardiac vessels were lifted and occluded by the device.

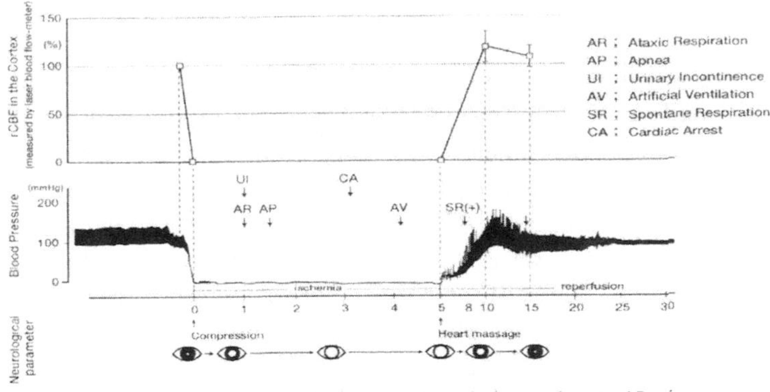

Physiological and Neurological parameters during and up to 15 min
after Compression of the major Cardiac vessels.

Fig. 4. Regional CBF (upper panel) and blood pressure (middle panel) recording during cardiac arrest and recirculation. Time course of the neurological parameters (middle and lower panels) during the operation. Physiological and neurological parameters during and up to 15 min after compression of the major cardiac vessels.

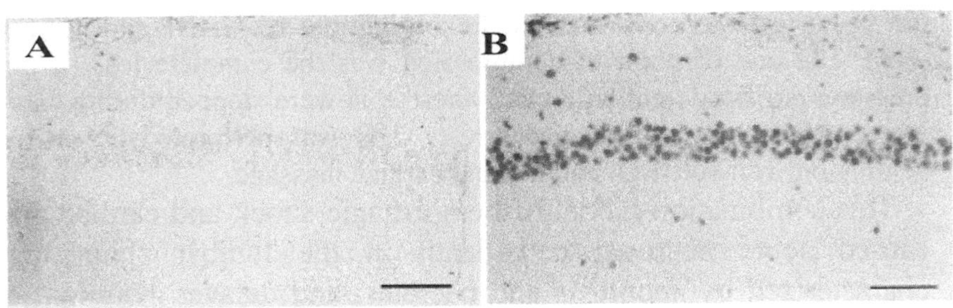

Fig. 5A, B. Staining of the rat hippocampus with the TUNEL method after ischemia. High-power fields of the sCA1 region (200x) showing 1 day (A) and 7 days (B) after ischemia. No TUNEL-positive pyramidal cells are visible in Day 1 (A). Numerous TUNEL-positive cells are visible 7 days after ischemia in the CA1 region. Scale bars: = 40 μm.

150

3.2 Cardiac arrest and hemorrhagic shock model (Kudo et al. 2006)

Recently, we developed a new rat model of whole body ischemia. This model was made by combining the cardiac arrest model and the 2VO + hypotension model. The ischemic intensity of this model is more severe than that of the cardiac arrest model. This model induces not only the degeneration of hippocampal CA1 regions but also the degeneration of the lumber spinal cord. Rats were intubated and anesthetized with inhalation of 2.0% sevoflurene, 70% N_2O in O_2. Rectal temperature was maintained at 37.0°C with a heat blanket. The left femoral artery and tail artery were dissected free and a polyethylene catheter (PE-50) was inserted for the withdrawal of arterial blood and for monitoring mean arterial blood pressure (MABP). During surgery, cardiac monitoring was performed using an ECG with subcutaneous needle electrodes.

After these procedures, heparin (100 U/Kg) was administered intra-arterially to avoid blood coagulation. Arterial blood samples were analyzed before ischemia and 10 min after resuscitation. Rats were administered 7 min of hemorrhagic shock and 5 min of cardiac arrest. Hemorrhagic shock was induced by withdrawing 3 ml/100 g arterial blood (Fig. 6). Resuscitation from hemorrhagic shock was performed by re-infusing the shed blood. In brief, the operator gently compressed the rat's chest with two fingers (index and middle) with force similar to that generated by a 3-kg weight, thereby inducing the cessation of ventilation. Cardiac arrest was confirmed by the diminutions of MABP and heart rate (HR). The end of point of compression was the complete loss of pulse pressure. Artificial ventilation and anesthesia were stopped during cardiac arrest. After 5 min of cardiac arrest, CPR was performed by artificial ventilation with 100% O_2 and manual cardiac massage.

This combination model of hemorrhagic shock and cardiac arrest caused acute neuronal cell death in the lumbar spinal cord, characterized by apoptosis and necrosis, and delayed neuronal cell death in the hippocampus, characterized by apoptosis.

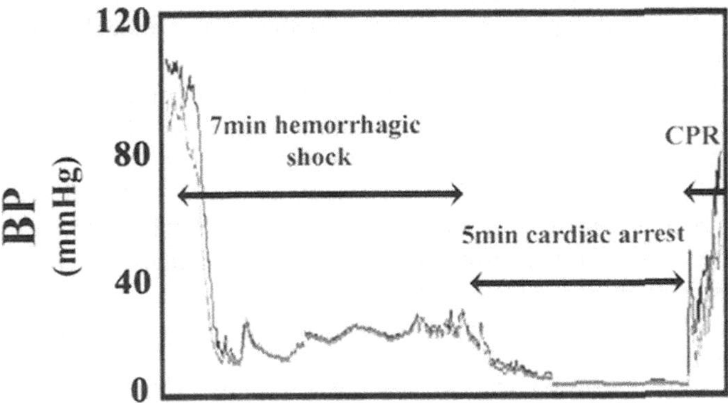

Fig. 6. Simultaneous recording of blood pressure (A). Withdrawal of arterial blood caused an initial drop (<20 mmHg) in blood pressure, followed by a second decrease (<10 mmHg) caused by chest compression (Kudo et al. 2006)

4 Conclusions

We have characterized the rat global ischemic models for the study of regeneration of CA1 pyramidal neurons. The models of forebrain ischemia are suitable for studies limited to brain ischemia. The models of forebrain ischemia are also simple, because there is no effect of the ischemic stress on other organs. On the other hand, the models of whole body ischemia are useful for the study of all organs including the brain and for inducing uniformity of the ischemia. However, the reaction to the brain ischemia may be influenced by the ischemic stress of the other organs in whole body ischemia models. There are many differences in the surgical procedures and a variety of drawbacks with each model. The appropriate model must be chosen on a study by study basis.

References

Beilharz EJ., Williams CE., Dragunow M., Sirimanne ES., and Gluckman PD. (1995) Mechanisms of delayed cell death following hypoxic-ischemic injury in the immature rat: evidence for apoptosis during selective neuronal loss. Brain Res Mol Brain Res 29, 1-14.
Bendel O, Bueters T, Euler M, Ogren AO, Sandin J, Euler G (2005) Reappearance

of hippocampal CA1 neurons after ischemia is associated with recovery of learning and memory. J Cereb Blood Flow Metab 25, 1586-1595.

Dohi K, Shioda S, Mizushima H, Homma H, Ozawa H, Nakai Y, Matsumoto K (1998) Delayed neuronal cell death and microglial cell reactivity in the CA1 region of the rat hippocampus in the cardiac arrest model. Med Electron Microsc 31, 85–93.

Hartman RE,T, Lee JM, Zipfel GJ, Wozniak DF (2005) Characterizing learning deficits and hippocampal neuron loss following transient global cerebral ischemia in rats. Brain Research 1043, 48–56.

Kawai K., Nitecka L., Ruetzler CA., Nagashima G., Joo F., Mies G., Nowak TS., Jr., Saito N., Lohr J. M., and Klatzo I. (1992) Global cerebral ischemia associated with cardiac arrest in the rat: I. Dynamics of early neuronal changes. J Cereb Blood Flow Metab 12, 238-249.

Kirino T. (1982) Delayed neuronal death in the gerbil hippocampus following ischemia. Brain Res 239, 57-69.

Koh JY, Suh SW, Gwag BJ, He YY, Hsu CY, Choi DW (1996) The role of zinc in selective neuronal death after transient global cerebral ischemia. Science 272, 1013–1016.

Korpatchev W, Lysenkov S, Thieliz P. (1982) Modielirowanlie klinczeskoj smerti l postreanimationznoj bolezni u krys. Palol Fiziol Exp Ter 3, 78-80.

Kudo Y, Ohtaki H, Dohi K, Yin L, Nakamachi T, Yofu S, Hiraizumi Y, Miyaoka H, Shioda S (2006) Neuronal damage in rat brain and spinal cord after cardiac arrest and massive hemorrhagic shock. Crit Care Medicine (in press)

Li. Y, Chopp M., Jiang N., Zhang Z., and Zaloga C. (1995) Induction of DNA fragmentation after 10 to 120 minutes of focal cerebral ischemia in rats. Stroke 26, 1252-1258.

MacManus JP., Buchan AM., Hill IE, Rasquinha I., and Preston E. (1993) Global ischemia can cause DNA fragmentation indicative of apoptosis in rat brain. Neurosci Lett 164, 89-92.

Nakatomi H, Kuriu T, Okabe S, Yamamoto S, Hatano O, Kawahara N, Tamura A, Kirino T, Nakafuku M. (2002) Regeneration of hippocampal pyramidal neurons after ischemic brain injury by recruitment of endogenous neural progenitors. Cell 110, 429–441.

Nitatori T., Sato N., Waguri S., Karasawa Y., Araki H., Shibanai K., Kominami E., and Uchiyama Y. (1995) Delayed neuronal death in the CA1 pyramidal cell layer of the gerbil hippocampus following transient ischemia is apoptosis. J Neurosci 15, 1001-1011.

Pulsinelli WA, Brierley JB (1979) A new model of bilateral hemispheric ischemia in the unanesthetized rat. Stroke 10, 267-272.

Wyllie AH., Kerr JF., and Currie AR. (1980) Cell death: the significance of apoptosis. Int Rev Cytol 68, 251-306.

Index

154

T